Concepts in community care for people with a learning difficulty

Edited by

P. Brigden & M. Todd

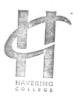

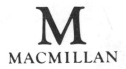

MACMILLAN

First published 1993 by
THE MACMILLAN PRESS LTD
Houndmills, Basingstoke, Hampshire RG21 2XS
and London
Companies and representatives
throughout the world

ISBN 0–333–57246–7

A catalogue record for this book is available
from the British Library

Printed in Hong Kong

Contents

iv · *Contents*

Contributors

Rosemary A. Baker MB, ChB, MRCGP, MRC Psych.
Consultant Psychiatrist in Mental Handicap, Priority Service Unit, Basingstoke, Hampshire

Patricia Brigden BSc, Dip. Clin. Psych., C. Psychol., Dip. Man. (OU)
Consultant Clinical Psychologist, East Berks Trust for People with Learning Difficulties, Bracknell, Berkshire

Caroline Carter BSc, MCSLT
Senior Speech and Language Therapist for people with learning difficulties, Priority Service Unit, Basingstoke, Hampshire

Tony Gilbert RNMH, BSc
Staff Development Officer, Tatchbury Mount Hospital, Southampton, Hampshire

Frances Loydd Dip. COT
Senior Occupational Therapist for people with learning difficulties and coordinator of a service for people with head injury, Priority Service Unit, Basingstoke, Hampshire

Julia Lloyd BSc, Dip. Clin. Psych.
Senior Clinical Psychologist, Priority Service Unit, Basingstoke, Hampshire

Steven Rose MSc, RNMH, RMN
Executive Director, Southwark Consortium for People with Learning Difficulties, Southwark, London

Tony Taylor RNMH, RMN, Qualified Psychotherapist
Locality manager and nurse psychotherapist for people with learning difficulties, Priority Service Unit, Basingstoke, Hampshire

Margaret Todd RNMH, RMN, RGN, Dip. N. (Lond.), FETC
Staff Development Manager, Priority Service Unit, Basingstoke, Hampshire

Jo Young RNMH
Clinical service manager for people with learning difficulties, Priority
Service Unit, Basingstoke, Hampshire

Heather Yule BA, MCFP
Manager of physiotherapy services for people with learning difficulties,
Priority Service Unit, Basingstoke, Hampshire

Introduction

Julia Lloyd

It is not the intention of this book to be the definitive text on the current and future provision of services for people with a learning difficulty. Many of the issues raised are more fully addressed in other texts. However, this book does provide an overview of the issues which affect the provision of services and provides some practical examples of how these could be incorporated into the reader's service. Whilst each chapter deals with a separate issue, there is cross referencing between chapters where appropriate to provide further clarification of the ideas explored.

Chapter 1 explores the social policy issues that have influenced the provision of care in this country over the past twenty years. In addition to this, the effects of the principles of normalisation are explored. This chapter also raises the issue that there is a wide variation in the definition of community facility. For example, Shalik & Shalik (1987) described the replacement of two large institutions by 26- and 24-place residences in America as a community facility. It is doubtful that these residences can be considered community facilities in this country.

In this book the term community facility is taken to mean residential units of eight places or fewer.

Chapter 2 explores the implementation of the new social policy in relation to service life cycles. The issue of what is a quality service and the notion of vision and guiding principles to be used for developing a quality service are examined. The importance of standards for all areas of service delivery is discussed. In addition to this, the comprehensiveness of standards, multidisciplinary team standards and quality assurance will be explored.

In order to implement a total quality management service it will be necessary to change some aspects of the service.

Chapter 3 identifies several change management strategies which may be useful to service planners and to hands-on care staff.

The issue of advocacy and self-advocacy is explored in Chapter 4. This leads on from Chapter 3, which indicates the need to ascertain the views and commitment of the clients of the service when implementing change strategies. Staff have tended to act as advocates to ensure that clients' rights are not violated and their needs are met. However, the extent to which they can do this is limited, and this is discussed fully in this chapter, as is the need to establish independent advocacy and self-advocacy schemes.

The closure of large, remote long-stay institutions for people with learning difficulties was promoted by a belief that living in the community would increase the quality of life experienced by these adults and children. The assumption was that by living in a family or in group homes, a person with a learning difficulty would automatically be provided with far greater opportunities for integration into community activities. Their proximity to local community affairs meant that opportunities to develop friendships with neighbours and other non-handicapped people would present themselves. It was hoped that community living would offer access to normal recreation facilities, such as hobbies, sports, restaurants, shops, and religious and political activities. The aim was that by locating family or group homes in residential areas, the close proximity to non-handicapped people that this offered would increase the contact between the two groups and that both groups would benefit. Chapter 5 explores how effective services have been in meeting these expectations, whilst Chapter 6 offers a practical approach to facilitating integration. The belief that moving people with learning difficulties to ordinary houses would increase their contact with non-disabled people is explored fully in Chapter 5 in terms of developing relationships. The development of relationships between people with a learning difficulty and non-handicapped individuals has not occurred to the extent that was envisaged. American research has indicated that, in terms of day-to-day contact, whilst people residing in group homes did go shopping, half of these people went shopping less than once a month (Crapps 1989), and thus their opportunity for community contact was not greatly enhanced.

People with learning difficulties may lead sheltered lives and engage predominantly in passive solitary leisure activities, such as watching television and listening to music. They have few friends outside their immediate families. The role of parents and carers in assisting social involvement therefore may be crucial. In a survey (McEvoy *et al*. 1990), it was found that only 28 per cent of people with a learning difficulty had been involved in local community clubs, and of these only one client still attended. Most parents felt that the local community was not sympathetic to them and said that they had to rely on service agencies. The survey also found that only 6 per cent of clients living at home had friends without a disability, although 75 per cent of parents wished for this to exist. This shows that although living in the community, many adults are still relatively isolated. This means that parents and carers need assistance to facilitate social contacts for this client group, as living in the community itself does not automatically provide integration. The ability of parents and carers to assist people with a learning difficulty in making friends becomes an important factor if community participation is to be anything more than an ideal. Chapter 6 provides useful practical guidelines on how to provide these clients with more challenging and valued leisure activities, which will assist in the achievement of community participation. Crapps (1989) found that the amount of community contact depended not only on the characteristics of the person with a learning difficulty, but also on the characteristics of the carer. This issue is also addressed in Chapter 6.

It is recognised that enabling people to live in ordinary houses and participate as fully as possible in the community is stressful. Whilst clients will be encouraged to use ordinary services, it is likely that they will also need specialist services. These may also include psychotherapy. The use of psychotherapeutic tools is a recent advance for this care group and Chapter 7 explores the efficiency and effectiveness of this approach.

Chapter 8 examines service provision from an individual perspective and addresses the issue of professional power in relation to achieving community participation and community presence and developing competence. Research indicates that relocating people into ordinary houses is not a significant factor in the development of social skills (McKay & Mackay 1989). Other research studies (Averno 1989) indicate that staff perceive that clients with learning difficulties participate less in community activities than a well integrated non-handicapped person. This indicates that living in ordinary houses alone does not ensure that people with learning difficulties will experience valued lifestyles, as discussed in Chapter 8. This chapter outlines various systematic approaches to care and provides an insight into the value base of these approaches. Shalik & Shalik (1987) described the difficulties these smaller institutions had in obtaining an adequate amount of occupational therapy services. This issue is addressed in Chapter 9. This chapter also explores the role of the physiotherapists and speech and language therapists in community-based services.

Chapter 10 continues the theme of ensuring that people with learning difficulties receive appropriate therapy, but this is from a medical perspective. This chapter addresses the issue of ensuring that the clients' ordinary and special medical needs are met in such a way as to promote their independence. The approach discussed incorporates the use of the multidisciplinary team to ensure that the care which the client receives is coordinated and meets his or her needs.

The final chapter addresses the issue of ensuring that the clients receive their care from a professional and skilled workforce. The issue of national vocational qualifications is addressed. In addition to this, a framework is provided which could be utilised to identify in a systematic way those skills that are required to deliver a quality service to the clients.

■ References

Averno, A. (1989). Community involvement of persons with severe retardation living in community residences. *Exceptional Children*. 55 (4), 309–14.

Crapps, J. (1989). Friendship patterns and community integration of family care residents. *Research in Developmental Disabilities*. 10, 153–69.

McEvoy, J., O'Mahoney, E. & Tierney, A. (1990). Parental attitudes and use of leisure by mentally handicapped persons in the community. *International Journal of Rehabilitation Research*. 13, 269–71.

McKay, T. & Mackay, D. (1989). Social skills of formally institutionalised mentally retarded persons. *Psychological Reports*. 64, 354.

Shalik, L. & Shalik, H. (1987). Cluster homes: A community for profoundly and severely retarded persons. *The American Journal of Occupational Therapy*. 41, 222–6.

Chapter 1

Social policy: a perspective on service developments and inter-agency working

Steven Rose

■ Introduction

Over the past two decades there have been significant changes in social policy towards people with learning difficulties. There are two types or levels of policy: first, 'official' social policy, which includes White Papers, government reports and enquiry findings; and second, 'unofficial' social policy, which includes a whole range of current concepts, examples of which are service brokerage, advocacy and normalisation. These various concepts have, over the years, influenced and shaped the way in which services have been delivered to people with learning difficulties. They make up what I refer to as 'secondary' social policy, are mainly transatlantic in origin, and have on the whole been far more influential in bringing about beneficial change, at the point of service delivery, than the major social policy documents and strategies of successive UK governments.

In fact, the official social policy of the last twenty years has, on the whole, been unsuccessful in making any significant impact on the lives of those with learning difficulties. For instance, in 1986, when the Audit Commission reviewed progress on the 1971 White Paper targets for people with learning difficulties, it found that only 39 per cent progress in the run-down of hospital places had been made towards the 1991 target (Table 1.1). To understand why, on the one hand, social policy has largely failed to bring about beneficial change, whilst on the other hand significant improvements in services have been brought about, it is necessary to understand the interrelationship between 'official' and 'unofficial' social policy. This interrelationship, together with other influences, such as the failure to achieve inter-agency working and the 'political' stances adopted by various professional groups, have all contributed to the slow rate of development over the years. Out of all of the unofficial social policy influences, the philosophy of normalisation (Wolfensberger 1972), and the principle of accomplishments

5

Table 1.1 Progress towards White Paper targets for mentally handicapped
people (England and Wales)

	1969	1984	Target (1991)	Progress to target
Hospitals (available beds – adults)	52 100	42 500	27 300	39%
Residential places (local authority, private and voluntary)	4 300	18 500	29 800	56%
Local Authority Adult Training Centre places	24 600	50 500	74 500	52%

Source: Audit Commission (1986)

(O'Brien 1986) have been the major contributors to guiding beneficial
change to services.

People with learning difficulties rely upon a range of agencies and
organisations to provide the services that they need. Traditionally these
services have been provided by the Departments of Education, Health,
Housing and Social Services as the main statutory agencies involved, with
some services being provided by the private and voluntary sectors. There
has been a lack of collaboration between agencies and organisations in key
areas such as planning, finance and staff training. Professional interests have
often overridden other issues and there has been a distinct lack of consumer
involvement in service planning and management.

Whilst various organisations and agencies are involved in service provision, coordination and inter-agency cooperation are essential for the
efficient and effective use of resources, ensuring that quality services are
experienced at the point of delivery. The history of inter-agency working,
against a background of the evolving social policy over the past twenty
years, is examined, along with some possible opportunities for change, in
the NHS and Community Care Act (Department of Health 1990).

In recent years the development of 'ordinary housing' schemes has been at
the centre of changes to service provision. The major 'unofficial' social policy
influence on service developments, and in particular, on the development of
housing schemes, has been the principle of normalisation; this principle also
transcends and encompasses the other concepts discussed, and hence it is the
main theme throughout this chapter. However, before looking at the effects of
the principle of normalisation on housing provision, it is important to consider
the development of current social policy in a historical context, and examine
the developments that have taken place in the twentieth century.

■ Official social policy in the twentieth century

People with learning difficulties were first recognised in law when the first Mental Deficiency Act of 1913 was passed; following the Act many of the existing institutions were developed through the 1920s and 1930s. Up until 1948 local authorities were the main statutory providers of services; although the private sector was also making a significant contribution at this time, most service provision consisted of institutional care. In 1948 with the creation of the National Health Service, the institutions were transferred to the new hospital authorities, and were the main resource of residential accommodation for all individuals with learning difficulties. In 1957 the situation was reviewed by a Royal Commission (DHSS 1957) which recommended major changes, including breaking down segregation and movement towards community care. This was followed by the 1959 Mental Health Act, which contained enabling legislation, the most significant change being that the majority of individuals were given 'informal' status, meaning that they were no longer certified and subject to detention in an institution. Thus the basic framework to enable community care to take place had been established.

Until the 1960s there had been little need for inter-agency working, as most services at that time were centred on health provision. This remained the case for severely handicapped children, who were excluded from the education system until April 1971. However, by 1971, the Departments of Health, Social Services, Housing and Education had become involved in service provision. In 1971 education was provided for children with learning difficulties by the local authority. Special schools were proposed in order to meet the children's educational needs. Until this time it was generally thought that these children were ineducable. These special schools enabled children who lived at home as well as those who resided in hospital to receive education. At this time a decade of public enquiries and scandals in the press concerning hospital services had begun (DHSS 1969; Martin 1986). Following each hospital scandal the government established a committee which was charged with the responsibility of determining the major factors which led to the scandal and for making recommendations to improve the service. The general findings of these committees predominately centred on overcrowded buildings, poor staffing levels, low staff morale, lack of privacy for clients, lack of activities for clients and the issue that clients generally received physical care only. The recommendations usually centred on enabling clients to have their own clothing, having adequate living space and receive some form of occupation and training. The government usually ensured that these hospitals received some extra funding to implement these recommendations (Martin 1986).

☐ **'Better Services for the Mentally Handicapped'**

It was against this background of changing philosophy towards community care, and an increasing number of public scandals surrounding existing services, that the government published the White Paper 'Better Services for the Mentally Handicapped' in June 1971 (DHSS 1971). It was noted that little or no progress had been made towards community care over the previous decade, that hospitals were overcrowded, buildings in need of repair or replacement, and that conditions were generally poor. The White Paper mapped out broad changes for the next twenty years that would shift the emphasis from hospital to community care. The targets set included the gradual run-down of hospital places, which was to be matched by a growth in local authority day and residential places. These changes would require close inter-agency working; in the words of the White Paper:

> The mentally handicapped and their families need help from professions working in services administered by a variety of authorities and departments. It is important that the resources of the health services, personal social services and education services should be deployed in close and effective collaboration. Only if this is done can the relevant professional skills be most effectively used to provide complete and co-ordinated services.

The need for inter-agency working, in terms of joint and coordinated planning, had been recognised. The White Paper had also recognised the importance of staff training, though had failed to make observations beyond the changes taking place within the training of nurses. The importance and potential of the emerging voluntary sector were also recognised. However, the White Paper failed to recognise the chasms between the cultures of the health and social services, the professional rivalry and in-fighting that was to emerge and the very real practical and structural barriers that existed, and largely continue to exist today, which hinder close inter-agency working. One of the best summaries of the factors which contribute to the imperfect state of inter-agency working is set out in Table 1.2, and was produced by the Working Group on Organisational and Management Problems of Mental Hospitals (DHSS 1979a).

If the forward-looking principles contained within the 1971 White Paper were to be translated into practice, then the structural issues, basic and post-basic training, issues of professionalism, and the concept of closer working with the voluntary sector would all have to be taken into account. In 1979 the structural issues had been clarified; however, no mechanisms had been developed to bridge the gap. There was a need for central leadership and direction to overcome the structural and cultural differences, to allow the pooling and sharing of resources and to cross the boundaries set up by differing conditions of employment in the various agencies. In addition to this, the financial implications of implementing the recommenda-

Table 1.2 Factors hindering effective inter-agency cooperation

National Health Service	Social Services Department
A chain of accountability to the DHSS	Largely controlled by locally elected representatives
Finance from the Exchequer	Substantial local funding
At local level management of services is separated from public accountability	Social Service Committee and Local Authority Members are responsible for management and public accountability
Geographical boundaries based on hospital services	Geographical boundaries based on local authorities
AHA (*now DHA / Self-governing trusts*) is a corporate/*independent* structure in itself	Social Service Committee is part of a corporate structure of a Local Authority
Dominant skills are clinical	Dominant skill is social work
A long history of training and expertise	Many untrained staff

tions of 'Better Services for the Mentally Handicapped' were never properly addressed.

☐ The 'Jay Report'

In 1975, under the Chairmanship of Mrs Peggy Jay, the Committee of Enquiry into Mental Handicap Nursing and Care was set up. Its task was to look at the staffing of mental handicap residential care in the NHS and local authorities. Part of its job was to look at the Briggs Committee's recommendation that 'a new caring profession for the mentally handicapped should emerge gradually' (DHSS 1972). The report of the committee (DHSS 1979b) was radical: it called for the move towards community care to be accelerated; for the number of care staff in the field to be doubled; and for management organisation to be streamlined; but for many, the most radical proposal of all was that the Central Council for Education and Training in Social Work (CCETSW) should be given the future responsibility for training all mental handicap residential care staff.

This final proposal evoked waves of indignant protest from nursing unions, health authorities, the General Nursing Council (GNC) and some parents' organisations. It brought about open hostility and contempt from mental handicap nursing staff towards colleagues in local authorities. At the time, it appeared that this report irrevocably damaged any chance that there ever was for collaborative inter-agency working.

However, at another level it can be argued that this radical social policy document helped bring about closer working between the agencies. After getting over the initial shock of being told that their skills were not necessarily relevant, the more forward-looking elements among mental handicap nurses set out to prove that they did have a role, and attempted to define their skill base. Whilst the motives of these nurses could be argued to be introspective and driven by self interest, this had the benefit of aiding inter-agency working and benefited individuals with learning difficulties.

There had been a rapid emergence of community mental handicap nurses in the second half of the 1970s (Hall & Russell 1980), with a growth from 16 community mental handicap nursing services in 1975 to 61 in 1979, employing over 200 nurses. This trend accelerated further after the publication of the Jay Report with over 400 trained nurses in post in the community by 1982 (Hall & Russell 1982). These nurses who were determined to prove their role started to work closely with other agencies and organisations, particularly through community mental handicap teams, so, whilst at a national level the debate raged on, there were many local examples of inter-agency working beginning to take place.

Another benefit to inter-agency working, which was a direct result of the Jay Report, was brought about by the GNC; following the publication of the Jay Report the GNC revised its syllabus of training for mental handicap nurses (GNC 1982). This revised syllabus shifted the emphasis of training from hospitals to the community, and nurses on placements increasingly worked alongside social workers, day centre staff, teachers and others.

There were further developments on the training front, post-Jay, which may be directly attributed to the policy document and enhanced inter-agency working. In the early 1980s there were several attempts to set up courses on either a joint or shared basis for Registered Nurses for the mentally handicapped students and Certificate in Social Services students. Although these early attempts achieved little in terms of establishing joint or shared training courses, at least the educationalists from different agencies were talking to each other. At a national level there was deadlock over the subject of basic training, with both the GNC and CCETSW unwilling to compromise. Some attempts to break the deadlock were made and various working parties and conferences were set up; however, there was little progress towards developing joint or shared basic training. The only result of two years of joint working between the General Nursing Council of the United Kingdom and CCETSW (GNC 1982) was to declare support in principle for the development of shared basic training. Joint training at both the qualifying and post-qualifying level appears to be an achievement of this working partnership in 1991.

□ Joint planning

The organisation required to coordinate and promote care in the community is fragmented between a number of statutory and voluntary agencies, and to overcome this problem the government introduced joint planning arrangements. Under Section 10 of the NHS Reorganisation Act (1973), a statutory obligation was laid upon health and local authorities to cooperate in respect of their individual functions. Health and local authorities were required to establish Joint Consultative Committees (JCCs), the function of which would be to advise 'on their performance in co-operative activities and on the planning and operation of services of common concern' (DHSS 1977).

In addition, health and local authorities were required to set up Joint Care Planning Teams at a local level under the general guidance of the JCC. In a further attempt to facilitate inter-agency working and joint planning, separate identified financial resources called 'joint finance' were made available to health authorities for spending specifically on joint schemes. In 1983, joint finance was extended to include education and housing. There were various restrictions on the uses to which joint finance could be put, though in essence joint finance was designed to allow the limited and controlled use of resources available to health authorities for the purpose of supporting selected personal social service spending by local authorities.

□ Joint finance

The introduction of obligatory joint planning mechanisms, and in particular joint finance, went some way towards facilitating inter-agency working. However, the procedures were cumbersome and bureaucratic, and owing to the frequent inability of local authorities to pick up the long-term revenue commitments of joint finance programmes, funds were often spent on health service projects, with the health authority picking up the revenue consequences. Joint finance has failed to make the impact on facilitating care in the community that it was originally hoped that it would.

Joint planning and a joint financial strategy have always been viewed as the key to successful inter-agency working. However, the major agencies involved in service provision have a consistently poor record of achievement in this area. When surveying District Health Authorities' planning groups (Wertheimer 1984) the Campaign for Mentally Handicapped People (CMH) recommended that

> If collaboration in planning is to become more effective, serious
> consideration must be given to how this can be achieved with
> agencies whose membership, planning cycles, and lines of
> accountability are different.

It also noted that

> If service planning is to move away from an almost total reliance on
> health and social services and towards the use of other provision
> such as ordinary housing stock and mainstream leisure facilities, it
> will be important for the providers of these services to be involved in
> the planning from an early stage.

A year later the Campaign for Mentally Handicapped People (now
Values into Action) pointed out (Wertheimer *et al.* 1985) that

> On the whole Regions were not involving local authorities in their
> planning activities to any significant degree

and that

> Agencies outside of the NHS are already major providers of services
> for mentally handicapped people. Local Authorities are at present the
> second biggest providers of services after the NHS. This provides a
> marked contrast to their general lack of involvement in Regional
> planning activities.

It may be seen that, in spite of clear policy guidelines from central
government, which had identified people with a learning difficulty as a
priority group (DHSS 1981), and the publication of various guidelines and
enabling policies (DHSS 1983; DHSS 1985; DHSS 1986a), that progress
towards inter-agency working had been slow. There remained problems at
an operational level and there was a clash of style and culture between
agencies. Perhaps the whole situation is best summed up by the following
quote from Mittler & Serpell (1985):

> In Britain, as in many other countries, relocation has been slow,
> partly because of the labyrinthine administrative and professional
> structures within which services are organised. These make it
> extraordinarily difficult to achieve coordination across service
> boundaries, and for professionals working in hospitals and local
> authorities to work together to achieve the discharge and
> rehabilitation of an individual resident.

By 1986 it had become clear that not only had the planning and
manpower aspects of inter-agency working on the whole failed to work, but
'a rationalisation of funding policies needed to be undertaken from the
centre so that the present policy conflicts could be resolved and the block
grant disincentives to the build-up of local authority community care ser-

vices removed' (Audit Commission 1986). The Audit Commission also suggested that local authorities could be made responsible for the long-term care of people with learning difficulties. The power to make payments towards community services, including the provision of housing by housing authorities and other bodies, such as housing associations and the Housing Corporation, was provided under the Health and Social Services and Social Security Adjudications Act (HMSO 1983). However, these discretionary powers were not being used on a wide basis. In spite of the fact that advocacy and self-advocacy had been established since 1968 (Williams & Shoultz 1982), little attention was given to these concepts in the 'official' policy publications of the mid-1980s. During this period the 1981 Education Act came into force. This enabled people with special educational needs to receive integrated education. Under the act all children who have special educational needs are to be assessed to ascertain what these needs are and how they can be met. The act also ensured that parents were fully involved in the assessment process. Another act which had the intention of involving clients in decisions about the services they receive is the 1986 Disabled Persons Act (DHSS 1986b). This act focuses on the rights of the individual. It attempts to give four rights: representation, assessment, information and consultation. However, only four sections of the act have been implemented to date. Section 3 of the act is in relation to assessment and requires Local Authorities to carry out a variety of assessments if requested to do so by the client. Following this, the Local Authority should provide a written statement stating what the individual's needs are (if any), and how these are to be met. If the needs are not to be met then the reason for this must be identified. Section 7 of the act requires Local Authorities to assess an individual prior to his or her discharge from hospital, providing the individual concerned does not object to this. Unfortunately, neither of these sections has been implemented.

The parts of the act that have been implemented are Sections 4, 8, 9 and 10. Section 4 requires local authorities to assess the needs of disabled people to ascertain whether they require services. Section 8 states that the local authorities should take into account the abilities of carers when assessing the need for services. Section 9 requires local authorities to inform people with disabilities of other organisations which offer services which may be relevant to their needs. Section 10 states that co-options or appointments to committees of people representing the interests of disabled people should only be made after consulting appropriate organisations of disabled people.

☐ **Care in the community: an agenda for action**

Following the publication of the Audit Commission report, the government asked Sir Roy Griffiths to undertake an overview of community care policy. The precise terms of reference were: 'To review the way in which public funds are used to support community care policy and to advise on the options for action that would improve the use of these funds as a contribution to more effective community care' (Griffiths 1988). When the report was finally published the main proposals were:

- a clearer strategic role for central government

- a more facilitative and enabling role for social services

- a better balance between policy aspirations and resources

- the creation of a ministerial post for community care

- continuing need for local collaboration between agencies

- new methods of financing community care

- a single gateway to publicly financed community care

- greater encouragement for a mixed economy of care

  Griffiths found a whole variety of agencies and organisations involved in community care, making effective inter-agency working almost impossible.

☐ Caring for people

Sixteen months after Sir Roy Griffiths produced what was a controversial report on community care, the government finally came up with its response. It had been widely rumoured for some time that at the highest of levels there was a great reluctance to accept the central proposal within the report: to give local authorities the lead responsibility for care in the community. The response was soon followed by a White Paper 'Caring for People' (Secretaries of State 1989).

It may be observed that there is something in the White Paper to appease all interested parties, thus: *The medical lobby* (para 2. 16): 'There will continue to be an important role for those such as consultants in the psychiatry of mental handicap'; *the nursing lobby* (para 2. 17): 'The mental handicap nursing profession plays a particularly important role in providing treatment, care and support to people with a mental handicap, both in hospital and a range of community settings'; *Local Authorities* (para 6.6): 'Social service authorities will be the "gatekeepers" to social care'; *the independent sector* (para 1.11): 'To promote the development of a flourishing independent sector . . .'; *the new right* (para 5.4): 'Where necessary, the government will not hesitate to intervene in order to stimulate improvements'; and the *residential care and the anti hospital closure lobby* (para 4.21): 'Health authorities will need to ensure that their plans allow for the provision of continuous residential health care for those highly dependent people who need it'.

The White Paper has been generally welcomed by Local Authorities, who see the lead agency role as a solution to many of the current inter-agency working problems. It remains to be seen whether there really is a rhetoric/reality gap, and if there are differences in the practicalities of implementation between the shires and inner cities.

The stated six key objectives of the White Paper are:

to promote the development of domiciliary and respite services to enable people to live in their own homes wherever feasible and sensible. Existing funding structures have worked against the development of such services. In future, the Government will encourage the targeting of home-based services on those people whose need for them is greatest;

to ensure that service providers make practical support for carers a high priority. Assessment of care needs should always take account of the needs of caring family, friends and neighbours;

to make proper assessment of need and good case management the cornerstone of high quality care. Packages of care should then be designed in line with individual needs and preferences;

to promote the development of a flourishing independent sector alongside good quality public services. The Government has endorsed Sir Roy Griffiths' recommendation that social service authorities should be 'enabling' agencies. It will be their responsibility to make maximum possible use of private and voluntary providers, and so increase the available range of options and widen consumer choice;

to clarify the responsibilities of agencies and so make it easier to hold them to account for their performance. The Government recognises that the present confusion has contributed to poor overall performance;

to secure better value for taxpayers' money by introducing a new funding structure for social care. The Government's aim is that social security provisions should not, as they do now, provide any incentive in favour of residential and nursing home care.

It could be suggested that there is a 'seventh' covertly stated key objective in the White Paper, which is 'to shut the gate on the rising annual cost of subsidising private residential care', which rose from £10 million to £1 billion in under a decade.

'Caring for People' received parliamentary assent in 1990, as part of The NHS and Community Care Act, and will be fully implemented in 1993. The NHS aspects of the act are being implemented in 1991, together with the requirement upon Local Authorities to draw up Community Care Plans. However, other demands, and in particular the implementation of the Children Act, have meant that the more important aspects of 'Caring for People', namely assessment, funding and care management will not be implemented until 1993.

To appreciate the implications of the act in terms of its potential to influence inter-agency working, it is necessary to look beyond its rhetoric to the opportunities that it presents to translate principles into practice. Social service departments will be the 'gatekeepers' to community care. However, there will remain areas where the distinctions between health and social care are blurred. Clarifying responsibilities in these areas will not be helped if various professional groups continue their fight for 'ownership' of people with learning difficulties. In 1990 the four Chief Nursing Officers of the United Kingdom commissioned a report on the skills of mental handicap nurses and their relevance in a mixed economy of care. The report, 'Mental Handicap Nursing In The Context Of Caring For People', was published in 1991. It introduced further new terminology: in referring to mental handicap nurses as being 'facility independent' it attempted to define the interface between health and social care in relation to people with learning difficulties, and to define some specific roles for the mental handicap nurse. Although 'Caring for People' has the potential to greatly influence inter-agency working, it may be observed that little has changed since the 1970s in terms of the tendency for professional interests to get in the way of inter-agency working.

There will be increased scope for the independent sector to respond imaginatively to the increased demand for individualised packages of care, and those in the public sector will increasingly have to become used to working with and alongside the independent sector. There will not be the same scope for fudging issues or avoiding joint working as there previously was. Local Authorities are now responsible for coordinating the production of Community Care Plans.

Market forces and contracts will increasingly ensure that services engage in inter-agency working. The voluntary and not-for-profit agencies have grown considerably over the past decade, and the scene is now set for these organisations to flourish. Contracts, new ways of directing benefits and case managers will ensure that these agencies are drawn centrally into the care delivery process.

Providing that funding responsibilities are kept separate, there is no reason why health and social services authorities cannot sell services to each other. The 'business' contract that will be involved in this process will prove to be a focus for inter-agency cooperation, and should assist in overcoming the problems associated previously with joint planning.

Joint planning has had limited success, and proposes to base future policy on planning agreements rather than joint plans. Unlike the previous joint planning arrangements, there are particular key requirements to joint planning agreements. The key requirements of planning agreements will be:

- common goals derived at least partly from national policy aims for particular client groups;

- funding agreements, setting out the basis on which health and social care will be funded;

- agreed policies on agreed operational areas, such as quality standards, assessment policies and procedures and discharge policies;

- agreed contract specifications for securing joint working between service providers.

The limited success of joint finance has been recognised and the government has announced its intention to review the future of this arrangement. The above approach is intended to achieve a shift in focus from means to ends, and if all else fails remember the ultimate sentence of (para 5.4) 'Where necessary, the Government will not hesitate to intervene in order to stimulate improvements'.

The language of 'Caring for People' may appear to be the vague and inexact language of persuasion that in the past has failed to bring about a workable joint planning process. It is repetitive and at times evasive; Chapter 6 on collaborative working ends with the sentence 'The Government will be giving further consideration to its future role in the light of wider changes'.

The White Paper, and the subsequent NHS and Community Care Act, did not go as far as the original Griffiths proposals, and to some extent it is a disappointing compromise in terms of bringing about inter-agency working. However, it does provide an opportunity to move firmly towards closer inter-agency working, that is if those at a local level are prepared to take radical steps, and move resolutely into uncharted territory, taking risks and putting aside old demarcation disputes. The announcement in 1990 that full implementation of 'Caring for People' will be delayed until 1993 came as a bitter blow to carers and those at the sharp end of service delivery in the community. However, this will at least give adequate time for proper joint strategies to be drawn up.

■ 'Unofficial' social policy

In the meantime, much service change is likely to be driven by what is referred to above as 'unofficial' social policy; this means the range of concepts and philosophies that have influenced service developments over the past two decades. Whilst these concepts all differ, they have one important factor in common, which is that they represent conceptual and practical means towards an acceptable quality of existence for those citizens within our society who have learning difficulties. The most recent arrival on the scene is 'service brokerage', whilst a constant influence on service provision over the past two decades has been the concept of 'normalisation'.

□ Normalisation

'Until about 1969, the term "Normalisation" had never been heard by most workers in social/health care. Today, it is a guiding principle standing for a whole new ideology of human management' (Wolfensberger 1972). The principle of normalisation originated in Denmark as early as 1959 and was actually written into Danish law governing services to the mentally retarded; in 1969 it was systematically stated in Swedish literature. In 1972 it was defined as follows: 'Utilization of means which are as culturally normative as possible' (Wolfensberger 1972). Normalisation is the oldest of the philosophies discussed and is actually a cornerstone of some of the other concepts. It is probably the most widely heard of philosophy and also the most widely misunderstood, though at the same time it is the most influential concept. It may seem strange that something can simultaneously be widely misunderstood and yet extremely influential; this needs some explanation.

Normalisation is a complex system which sets out to value positively devalued individuals and groups, and is influential at three levels. These levels are a personal level, primary and intermediate social systems and a societal level.

The language and terminology of normalisation are North American and the evaluation system/process is complex (Wolfensberger & Glenn 1975). The use of the evaluation system 'Programmed Assessment of Service Systems' requires considerable training, and the language and terminology is often incomprehensible, even to those already involved in services for people with learning difficulties. Few really appreciate the corollaries and implications of the normalisation principle. Also, probably because of the vague nature of the word, it has often been used by those who either do not understand it, or choose deliberately to misinterpret it to justify a whole range of misdeeds and poor services. Hence the most influential concept ever with regard to services for people with learning difficulties unfortunately remains misunderstood and misapplied in many circumstances. However, one has to look no further than the set of service principles that govern many services throughout health services, local authority services and the voluntary sector to see evidence of the far-reaching effect of the principle of normalisation.

☐ **Accomplishments**

The concept of 'accomplishments' as a measure and standard around which to base services arrived in the mid-1980s (O'Brien 1986). These simple but powerful statements have produced significant beneficial and ongoing changes to some services in their capacity as 'unofficial' social policy. The accomplishments are: Dignity and Respect, Community Presence, Community Participation, Choice and Competence.

An example of accomplishments being adapted to form service principles is set out below (Southwark Consortium 1991):

Dignity and Respect People with a learning difficulty have the right to be treated with respect and dignity. They will be offered services which are based on their individual circumstances, choices and expectations; they will participate in decision making; they will be given information; they will have the right of refusal and complaint through self advocacy and advocacy; and will be involved in developing and evaluating the services they receive. People will have services which are appropriate to their age and which they can be proud of.

Community Presence People with a learning difficulty are part of the community and must not be separated from it; they will have equal opportunities in having easy access to shops, leisure and recreation, housing, education, employment, Health Services, Social Services, etc.

Community Participation People with a learning difficulty must be able to develop a full range of personal relationships; to be involved with others as friends, relatives, colleagues, consumers and citizens; and to have sexual relationships and options which include marriage and parenting.

Choice People with a learning difficulty have the right to make choices and decisions about their daily lives and activities, and to be enabled to make choices and decisions with support and information about options, responsibilities and consequences. People with a learning difficulty have the right to services which promote the taking of risks and the holding of personal options.

Competence People with a learning difficulty will have opportunities to develop skills through their lives by building on their skills and abilities in a variety of settings with a variety of means to enable them to be involved in the community.

☐ Housing

Housing is a crucial component of community care. It is of fundamental importance to all individuals, central to quality of life, and, if inadequate, it has serious detrimental effects on mental and physical well-being. Incorporated within service principles which are based on normalisation will be principles relating to housing, an example being:

> Our goal is to see mentally handicapped people in the mainstream of life, living in ordinary houses, in ordinary streets, with the same range of choices as any citizen, and mixing as equals with the other, and mostly not handicapped members of their own community (King's Fund 1980).

In many areas this principle is being translated into practice, as the residential services are developed in ordinary housing.

A brief examination of the range of services provided by various organisations soon indicates that there exists a wide interpretation of what the term 'ordinary housing' can mean. It is not uncommon to find 25-bed hostels masquerading as community homes, and presented as examples of 'normalised' living. Another common model of so called ordinary housing is one where eight people will be found living together; this size of model has become particularly popular with many organisations. The reason for the popularity of the eight-place model is simple: it is large enough for the residents to attract maximum DSS benefits, whilst small enough to be economically staffed and stake a claim to be a model of 'ordinary'/ 'normalised' living.

In many areas the maximum size of house being developed has three places. Often, a group of three people living together is the maximum number that will allow any degree of 'ordinary living'. It is not coincidental that larger groups fall within the requirements of the 1984 Registered Homes Act. In the quest towards normalisation, service planners have been tied to the idea that small equals normalisation. There is certainly some merit in the idea, as there is at least a chance of putting the principles of normalisation into practice in a three- or four-place house, whilst there is no chance in the old large hospital wards, or in the modern 25-place units. There are other important ingredients to normalised housing, which include proper identification of individual needs, choice and empowerment.

It is easy to criticise the housing provided when it is measured against the principles of normalisation; however there are many practical constraints upon providing housing for people with learning difficulties. This often means that while philosophies, plans and developments are driven by the principle of normalisation, there are compromises made on the way, and the final development falls short of the principles of normalisation.

☐ Legislation and normalisation

Legislation can often hinder normalised housing developments. Changes to the Town and Country Planning Act in 1987 meant that planning permission from Local Authorities was no longer required for developments of up to six places. This should be viewed as a significant move forward for the principle of normalisation, as it affects housing. However, while government may have taken a step in the right direction regarding planning regulations, departmental guidelines on fire precautions, with which Health and Local Authorities and the voluntary and private sectors must comply, have not incorporated the principles of normalisation. Guidelines on fire precautions are contained within the Government Circular HN (85) 33, with HTM 88 appended, and stipulate such requirements as enclosed stairwells, exit signs, smoke detectors, half-hour fire resistant doors, and fire extinguishers. Whilst all of these precautions and the others contained within the guidelines may be considered laudable in themselves, they do place constraints on aspects of normalisation.

One Health Authority discovered that two of its group homes fell far short of the majority of the regulations contained within HTM 88, and, due to the particular construction of the buildings in question could not readily bring them up to standard. A formal decision was eventually taken to ignore some aspects of the departmental guidelines on fire precautions. The basis upon which this decision was made was that the clients had lived in the houses for several years and that they were happy, well integrated and did not wish to move. Additionally, they had a level of staff support linked to their identified needs and wants, and all the precautions that were possible had been carried out. Incidentally, the two houses concerned formed part of a terrace of council houses occupied by ordinary families, who were in just as much 'danger' from fire as the people with learning difficulties in the Health Authority group homes. This was truly an example of 'people with a learning difficulty, in the mainstream of life, living in ordinary houses, in ordinary streets, with the same range of choices as any citizen, and mixing as equals with other, and mostly not handicapped members of their own community' (Kings Fund 1980). However, these types of decision are rarely made by Health Authorities or Social Service Committees; it is a brave and forward thinking authority that is prepared to take up this stance on behalf of people with learning difficulties.

☐ Evaluation of housing

There now exist a whole range of housing schemes for individuals with learning difficulties, administered by Local Authorities, Health Authorities, voluntary organisations and charitable trusts. The various schemes are well described elsewhere by others, (Towell 1988; Shearer 1986; Felce 1988;

Thomas *et al.* 1978). In the past much of the work published concerning housing schemes has tended to be descriptive rather than evaluative, and many of the authors have described services that they have been associated with rather than seeking external evaluation.

More recently, work of a far more evaluative nature has begun to emerge. Booth *et al.* (1989) completed a major survey of independent living schemes, covering 149 schemes accommodating 349 people in four different parts of the country. This study takes a wide look at independent living schemes, at the type and range of accommodation provided, and attempts to piece together a profile of the characteristics of the people living within the various schemes. The study concluded that although there was a high rate of placement success, it remained to be seen whether this would be continued in the long term, when longitudinal data becomes available. Twenty nine per cent of the people in the survey had moved direct from hospital. Over half had spent some time in hospital, and a quarter had lived in hospital for over fifteen years. These figures are a clear demonstration of the principle of normalisation being applied at the level of primary and intermediate social systems, and having already taken effect at a societal level, in so far as it has shaped the policy which has led to this type of development.

However, it would be a mistake to assume that the effects of normalisation in influencing beneficial change at higher levels are necessarily transmitted to a personal level in independent and ordinary housing schemes for people with learning difficulties. Correct principles and philosophy together with ordinary housing do not always lead to a normalised existence at a personal level. There are other important ingredients. To measure the influence of normalisation on housing at a personal level it is necessary for careful and close evaluation of the individual's life to take place, for aspects of quality to be measured, and for account to be taken of the interaction between normalisation and other concepts and systems in operation.

Bratt & Johnson (1988) look at the quality of life of five young people after they left hospital to live in a bungalow in Exeter. They found a number of indications consistent with the view that the quality of life of the young people had improved as a result of leaving hospital. The individuals went out more, and to more varied places; they spent more time engaged in interaction with other people; and less behaviour judged to be 'inappropriate' was recorded. On the other hand they found little evidence of integration being achieved within the local community; and there was no evidence of individuals being supported in ways which increased their competence, particularly in relation to participation at a simple level in doing routine domestic tasks. Bratt and Johnson noted that these findings were in contrast to those of previous researchers (Mansell *et al.* 1984; Thomas *et al.* 1986). This is interesting in itself, as the majority of published research into ordinary housing does tend to dwell on the more positive findings. They went on to say that whilst the project had created an improved quality of life, it had failed so far to exploit many of the opportunities available for changing life styles. Finally, they said that there needs to be a clear statement by the authority responsible for the housing development regarding the explicit changes in life style being sought. Such statements they said 'need to be explicit and to go beyond obtuse ambitions' (for example, 'respecting individual needs', 'following the principle of normalisation', 'integration') unless they are subsequently translated into more specific guidance. It is reasonable to conclude that, as indicated above, the principle of normalisation alone has not been entirely successful in producing normalised living and housing. Additional systems and concepts need to be introduced with it at an interactional level to ensure that the principle is translated into practice at a personal level with regard to housing for people with learning difficulties.

☐ Service brokerage

During the past few years, in Canada the concept of 'service brokerage' has emerged: empowering individuals with learning difficulties to have control over their own lives is at the heart of this concept. This has coincided with changes to the law (in the Charter of Rights and Freedoms, and in the extension of human rights legislation). There have been subsequent changes in policy, public attitudes and expectations of social and human services. Service brokerage is a unique concept which was designed by parents of individuals with learning difficulties. The fundamental starting point of the concept is a recognition that if society really wants to empower disabled individuals, so that they can live full lives as equal members of society, then some critically important links missing from our present social service systems need to be installed.

Brokerage is but one part of a three-dimensional 'support nucleus' which consists of:

(a) the personal network;

(b) individualised funding which ties monies to the individual;

(c) an autonomous planning vehicle, acting as a fixed point of responsibility and planning and providing service brokerage as required to the individual who is supported by his or her personal network.

Service brokerage is the technical arm of the autonomous and individualised planning service, and only when all three components are in place can the brokerage element work. The three components allow the broker to ensure that the individual has access to services on the open market, purchasing those required. Funding is always allocated to the individual, who supported by his or her personal network, controls the planning, decision making and service purchasing process. With a service brokerage system in operation, there is no longer any need for statutory agencies to be involved in the service planning process or service provision.

This sort of system has yet to make any impact on services within the United Kingdom. However, its potential is enormous, and such a system would override and circumvent the issues and problems around inter-agency working. There are almost certainly prerequisites to establishing such a system within the UK, and one of these is the further development of advocacy and self-advocacy (see Chapter 4).

Additionally, new ways of working together by statutory agencies, voluntary organisations, consumers and their representatives need to be found.

■ Conclusion

The NHS and Community Care Act is now with us, and in the process of being implemented. It will bring fundamental changes to the way in which services are to be funded. There will be a single budget under the control of local authorities to cover the cost of community care. Most local authorities are now establishing a 'case management' approach. Case management, whilst representing a significant step forward from the way that most services are provided at present, is not service brokerage. The main change in the provision of housing for those people with learning difficulties who have been fortunate enough to leave hospital is that they now live in smaller units of accommodation, based within the community. They have yet to experience all aspects of normalised living.

Service brokerage, a system that is working well in Canada, represents a way forward which can bring about truly needs-led and individualised services (*Community Living* 1989). A case management approach would represent only a partial step forward, though it may be necessary to take this evolutionary step to reach the ultimate goal.

Over the past fifteen years a whole range of concepts have influenced the provision of services for people with learning difficulties. Care in the community has been a central theme throughout that period, though progress has been slow and sporadic. Political commitment and the will to translate central policy into practice at a local level are essential ingredients in successfully providing services in ordinary settings.

The philosophy of normalisation continues to be our guiding star, though there have been misunderstandings and many obstacles in the way over the years, and the principles contained within accomplishments are providing the means to put philosophies into practice.

The most exciting concept to appear for many years is service broker-age; and it may eventually radically alter the current systems of service provision in the United Kingdom. It represents a real opportunity to hand over power to the consumer (Brandon & Towe 1989).

A model to achieve integrated services at a local level can be achieved through the formation of consortia. This involves health authorities, social services departments, housing associations, adult education and a range of local voluntary organisations pooling resources into a consortium, for the purpose of service provision and planning. Consumers can be fully involved in running these services, and the independent sector made wide use of through the process of contracting.

The first consortium was formed in 1984 (Southwark Consortium 1991), and now functions on behalf of two Health Authorities, the Local Authority and a variety of other organisations; it manages 150 places in 37 properties, and a range of other services. Currently there is a small but gradual growth in the formation of consortia in response to the NHS and Community Care Act.

There is nothing within the Act which will preclude this from happening, though such simple innovation still goes beyond the imagination of many health and local authorities. There is scope for both authorities to retain their statutory responsibilities, including local authorities' responsibilities of assessment and 'gatekeepers' to social care, through the purchaser and provider split. Such a step goes beyond the level of inter-agency working hinted at within the White Paper. Professional differences have to be put aside, however, so that the expertise of professional inputs can be maintained. It is to be hoped that more enlightened authorities will rise to this challenge, and adopt an approach which incorporates the concepts of normalisation and service brokerage.

In May 1991 the government announced that the term 'mental handicap' is to be replaced by the term 'people with learning disabilities'. This was widely accepted as a significant step forward; even though the term 'learning difficulties' which the people who have to carry the label say they would prefer (Values into Action 1991) was not chosen. In the same announcement Stephen Dorrell, the Health Minister, indicated that there was a place for care villages alongside community care. This came as a bitter blow for those who have been campaigning for the closure of institutions over many years.

This latter announcement has led to a joint initiative by the Royal College of Nursing and Values into Action to form The Coalition for Community Care for People with Learning Difficulties. The Coalition has over a dozen member organisations, including advocacy organisations, national charities, campaigning organisations, professional organisations and a health service trade union. Some onlookers have been bewildered by a coalition of organisations with such publicly different agendas; however, such working together will bring benefits to people with a learning difficulty.

The past two decades have seen the exposure of terrible services, ideas and commitment to change, resistance and professional rivalry, and inadequate central coordination of planning and funding. This has meant that 'official' social policy has largely failed to bring about the desired changes. In spite of this, 'unofficial' social policy has helped steer and develop service provision in the desired direction. The latest government announcements are both heartening and concerning at the same time.

■ References

Audit Commission (1986). *Making a reality of community care*. HMSO, London.
Audit Commission (1989). Developing community care for adults with a mental handicap, *Occasional Papers*. HMSO, London.
Booth, T., Phillips, D., Berry, S., Jones, D., Lee, M., Mathews, J., Melotte, C., & Pritlove, J. (1989). Home from home: a survey of independent living schemes for people with mental handicaps. *Mental Handicap Research*, 2:2, 152–6.
Brandon, D. & Towe, N. (1989). *Free to choose. An introduction to Service Brokerage*. Good Impressions Publishing, London.
Bratt, A. & Johnson, R. (1988). Changes in life style for young adults with profound handicaps following discharge from hospital care into a 'second generation' housing project. *Mental Handicap Research*, 1:1, 49–74.
Community Living (1989). Supplement: *How Service Brokerage works*. April 1989, p. i–viii. Good Impressions Publishing, London.
Department of Health (1990). *The NHS and Community Care Act 1990*. HMSO, London.
DHSS (1957). *Report of the Royal Commission on the law relating to mental illness and mental deficiency*, 1954–57. Cmnd 169. HMSO, London.
DHSS (1969). *Report of the committee of inquiry into allegations of ill-treatment of patients and other irregularities at Ely Hospital, Cardiff*. Cmnd 3975. HMSO, London.
DHSS (1971). *Better services for the mentally handicapped*, Cmnd 4683. HMSO, London.
DHSS (1972). *Report of the Committee on Nursing*. Cmnd 5115. HMSO, London.
DHSS (1977). *Joint care planning: Health and Local Authorities*. Circular HC (77) 17/LAC (77) 20. HMSO, London.
DHSS (1979a). *Organisational and management problems of mental illness hospitals*. HMSO, London.
DHSS (1979b). *Report of the committee of enquiry into mental handicap nursing and care*. HN (79) 27 Cmnd 7468. HMSO, London.
DHSS (1981). *Care in action: A handbook of policies and priorities for health and personal social services in England*. HMSO, London.
DHSS (1983). *Health Service development: care in the community and social finance*. Circular HC (83) 6/LAC (83)5. HMSO, London.
DHSS (1985). *Government response to the second report from the Social Services Committee 1984–5 session*. Cmnd 9674. HMSO, London.
DHSS (1986a). Collaboration between the NHS, Local Government and

Voluntary Organisations: Joint planning and collaboration. *Draft Circular.* HMSO, London.

DHSS (1986b). *The Disabled Persons (Services, Consultation and Representation) Act 1986.* HMSO, London.

Felce, D. (1988). *The Andover Project: staffed housing for adults with severe or profound mental handicaps.* BIMH Publications, Kidderminster.

GNC (1982). *Training syllabus for Registered Nurses for mental subnormality nursing.* General Nursing Council for England and Wales, London.

Griffiths, Sir Roy (1988). *Community care: Agenda for action,* HMSO, London.

Hall, V. & Russell, O. (1980). A national survey of community nursing services for the mentally handicapped. *Mental Handicap Studies Research Report No. 10,* University of Bristol, Department of Mental Health, Bristol.

Hall, V. & Russell, O. (1982). The community mental health nurse: A new professional role. *Research Report* No. 11. University of Bristol, Bristol.

Health and Social Services and Social Security Ajudications Act (1983). HMSO, London.

King's Fund (1980). *An ordinary life.* King Edward's Hospital Fund for London.

Mansell, J., Jenkins, J., Felce, D. & De Kock, U. (1984). Measuring the activity of profoundly and severely mentally handicapped adults in ordinary housing. *Behaviour Research and Therapy,* **22,** 23–9.

Martin J. (1986). *Hospitals in trouble.* Blackwell, Oxford.

Mittler, P. & Serpell, R. (1985). Services: an international perspective. In A. M. Clarke, D. B. Clarke, & J. M. Berg (eds): *Mental deficiency: The changing outlook.* 4th edn. Methuen, London.

O'Brien, J. (1986). A guide to personal futures planning. In G. T. Bellamy, & B. Wilcox (eds): *The activities catalogue.* Responsive Systems Associates, Georgia, USA.

Secretaries of State for Health and Social Security, England, Wales and Scotland (1989). *Caring for people: Community care in the next decade and beyond.* HMSO, London.

Shearer, A. (1986). *Building community.* Campaign for People with Mental Handicaps & King Edward's Hospital Fund for London.

Southwark Consortium for people with learning difficulties (1991). *Information package.* 27 Barry Road, London.

Thomas, D., Firth, H. & Kendall, A. (1978). *ENCOR – A way ahead.* CMH Publications, London.

Thomas, M., Felce, D., De Kock, U., Saxby, H. & Repp, A. (1986). The activity of staff and of severely and profoundly mentally handicapped adults in residential settings of different sizes. *British Journal of Mental Subnormality,* **32,** 82–92.

Towell, D. (1988). *An ordinary life practice: Developing comprehensive community based services for people with learning disabilities,* King Edward's Hospital Fund for London.

Values into Action (1991). *The newsletter of the national campaign with people who have learning difficulties.* Issue No 65, Summer 1991.

Wertheimer, A. (1984). *A survey of District Health Authorities' planning groups for services to people with mental handicaps.* CMH Publications, London.

Wertheimer, A., Ineichen, B. & Bosanquet, N. (1985). *Planning for a change: A*

study of Regional Health Authorities' planning of services for people with mental handicaps. CMH Publications, London.
Williams, P. & Shoultz, B. (1982). *We can speak for Ourselves: Self Advocacy by mentally handicapped people.* Indiana University Press, Bloomington.
Wolfensberger, W. (1972). *Normalisation: The principle of normalisation in human services.* p. 27. National Institute of Mental Retardation, Toronto.
Wolfensberger, W. & Glenn, L. (1975). *PASS 3, Program Analysis of Service Systems.* National Institute of Mental Retardation, Toronto.

Chapter 2

Quality issues

Patricia Brigden and Margaret Todd

■ Introduction

The National Health Service and Community Care Act 1990 (Department of Health 1990a) looks certain to bring about the most dramatic reorganisation the National Health Service has seen since its inception in 1948. It aims to create an internal market with the express intention thereby of improving both its efficiency and its effectiveness. Just as the arrival of the single European market in 1993 will increase competitiveness, so that companies who want to remain competitive will have to prepare and train staff to meet this competition, provider units will also have to sharpen up their performance to stay in business in the new market environment of the National Health Service. It has been stated that quality has little value other than having an essential part to play in improving the competitive edge. It is argued here, however, that even in these financially conscious times it is the single most important consideration for a service where the principle aim is to provide quality care.

Many definitions of quality exist. It has been stated that quality is a dynamic process. Historically, quality has meant compliance with minimal standards such as adequate space and minimal staffing levels. The concept of quality in today's service can be perceived as a degree of excellence (Wieck *et al.* 1989). Quality is what the customer wants. It is determined by the customer. It is measured against customer requirements, either stated or perceived, and consequently it is always changing in a competitive market place.

British Standard 4778 (1987) defines quality as the 'Totality of features and characteristics of a product or service that bear on its ability to satisfy stated or implied needs'. The benefits of a quality service are a service which meets the customer's expectations or requirements. It ensures value for money because procedures and processes are soundly based and efficient, reducing errors and ensuring the efficient deployment of resources. A quality service ensures that there are well-documented records which assist in making service changes and improvements. The documentation ensures that there is a complete record of every aspect of service provision and this can be controlled throughout the process of change and improvement. A common understanding of the organisation's quality policies, aims and objectives is essential, and it is important that all staff within the organisation have the same shared vision of what is a quality life for clients.

A quality organisation is customer-led; that is it provides what the client needs and it delivers the service in accordance with the client's wishes. The individual is of central importance and the services are delivered to meet individual clients' needs. This approach is currently enshrined in the government paper 'Caring for People' (Department of Health 1990b). A quality service delivers only as much help as is needed by the client and no more. The utilisation of this approach should contain costs, as it enables available resources to be matched against clients' actual needs and over-provision or duplication of services should be eradicated.

Another aspect of a quality service is that it values people, and it has the same value base for both clients and staff. The goals of the organisation are shared with service users and staff and are subsequently influenced and shaped by these key people. Managers of the service use the complaints procedure as an opportunity to learn about service defects and take appropriate actions to rectify these. As such, a quality service is always seeking ways to improve the standards of care it offers.

Since meeting customer requirements in full is an important aspect of what is meant by quality, a first consideration has to be: 'Who is the customer?'. It is worth thinking about the concept that in any organisation there are internal customers and suppliers, such as a manager and his or her secretary. The secretary supplies typed letters for the manager, and is the supplier whilst the manager is the customer. If the secretary supplies error-free work, on time and laid out as the manager wishes, then the manager is a satisfied customer. Conversely if the secretary cannot read the manager's writing then he or she cannot work properly and the work may have to be redone, at additional cost to the company. These examples are given to illustrate the fact that the 'customer' in a business sense means far more than the client and/or carers. Indeed, the District Health Authority will become a customer as it purchases services from provider units and it will want to ensure that the service it purchases is of an adequate standard and provides value for money.

■ Total quality management

Several factors have been identified as contributing to good quality. These are: good service design to meet clients' needs; clients must be able to rely on the service being provided when it is needed; it must be at the correct price; and the service must be cost-effective. The concept of quality can be examined in a variety of ways. The issues which will be explored here are:

- Total quality management.
- Working practices.
- Client outcomes.
- Quality assurance tools. Audit is one of many possible methods of measuring quality.

The principles of total quality management are:

- Putting the client/carers first.
- Being fully aware of the clients' expectations and needs.
- Satisfying each client's needs and satisfying them first time.
- Recognising the cost of poor quality, such as clients not using the service in the future and bad publicity resulting from a poor quality service.
- Supporting and encouraging every member of staff in every setting: staff must feel as valued as clients.
- Encouraging staff loyalty to their workplace and employer.
- Encouraging enthusiasm, knowledge and skills in staff to help them deliver higher quality care and cost-effective health care services.
- Encouraging professionalism and expertise among all staff.

Total quality management can be represented diagrammatically, as in Figure 2.1. Thus it can be seen that total quality management includes organisational quality, customer quality and professional quality.

Organisational quality involves the mission statement of the provider unit and how the service components fit in with this. The mission statement indicates the values, beliefs and purpose of the provider unit, and the philosophy of the service for people with learning difficulties should relate to this overall mission statement. Formal or structured ways in which members of staff and clients are involved in influencing the service and quality issues should exist or be established as a matter of urgency. The consumers' views are required at every level of the service, as it is their needs which the service is required to meet. If they do not have a voice to the higher echelons of service providers, how can the service be certain that its plans and delivery of service meet the customers' expectations? (See Chapter 4 for information regarding advocacy and citizen advocacy.) Systems to gather customers' views should be introduced at the design and manage-

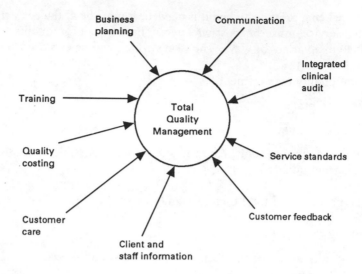

Figure 2.1 The elements of total quality management.

ment level of the service. Managers of the service should actively pursue methods of improving relationships with service users, their carers and advocates. The complaints procedure can be utilised in this way if customers see that their complaints are treated seriously and sensitively, and that resultant action is taken to rectify the situation from which the complaint arose, without detrimental effects for the complainant.

The issue of professional quality includes acceptance of professional standards relating to national guidelines which exist for many groups of staff (such as physiotherapists), and how these are being used in practice. Staff should be working to an agreed level of individual professional standards, and systematic processes for monitoring achievements, such as peer review, should exist. Whilst this at first sight may appear threatening to individual staff members, it has been found that the majority of people favour peer review as a valuable method of receiving feedback on their performance. This needs to be handled sensitively and should focus on the good performances of the individual as well as on what performances they need to improve.

■ Quality strategy

Services should have a quality strategy. This involves:

● creating procedures to meet quality standards;

- communicating standards and procedures to employees and training them to action these;

- monitoring and controlling standards;

- delivering a quality programme, which includes:
  - obtaining organisational commitment
  - agreeing a common mission
  - opening and maintaining communication.

These aspects of a quality programme need further consideration.

☐ Mission statements, goals and objectives

The mission statement is a statement in writing describing the fundamental reason for the organisation's existence. It sets out beliefs and responsibilities, describes the general scope of activities and defines the users. It should be regularly reviewed, as it needs to be altered as circumstances change. Goals are statements about activities needed to achieve the mission. They are expressed in a way that makes it easy to see if they have been achieved. Objectives are clear, precise statements of parts of the goal. They can be measured. They describe outcomes, not processes. To help individual units of a service decide on goals and objectives it is necessary to identify valued features of the service which would be crucial to user satisfaction.

☐ Indicators

Indicators are criteria by which a standard is judged. A standard is a level of service which should be achieved. Quality improvement techniques are a variety of methods and accompanying problem solving techniques which can be introduced to facilitate the quality process. Some sort of reporting system is necessary to keep a track of progress. An example from the field of learning difficulty can be seen in the Portage service, a home teaching service for preschool children with learning difficulties. The *goal* is to teach children skills based on an assessment of their needs. The *objective* is to set three to six activity charts for parents to complete each week. The *feature* indicating evidence of progress is learning of skills by the child. The *indicator* is percentage of completed activity charts which can be achieved. The *monitor* is weekly audit at team meetings. The standard is 88 per cent successful achievement of the skills by the child as evidenced by completion of the activity charts. Quality improvement techniques include direct feedback to teachers and parents, coaching from supervisors or visiting experts, and staff training.

☐ **Standards**

Little can be achieved until agreement has been reached as to standards (where standards represent the level of service which should either be aimed at or achieved). The first critically important consideration has to be the point at which standard of care becomes unacceptably low. While people agree that care practices described in some settings, such as parts of Romania and the Greek island of Leros are unacceptable, there is a middle range of care where public opinions tend to differ. Thus, for example, a 30-bed single-sex ward would be considered inadequate in some parts of the United Kingdom, yet in others it would be tolerated, ostensibly because of resource restrictions (also possibly because of lack of commitment or lack of belief in the desirability of community care). In order not to demoralise those who have to work in areas where the organisation's standards of care are less than the ideal, such as where large hospital wards still of necessity exist, it is worth pointing out that the object of the exercise is to give the best quality of care that one can, given current resources. This is necessary, as in some situations real changes to achieve the ideal may take ten years' planning time. Perhaps the first measure of quality that should be considered in looking at any organisation should be to ask whether it has an agreed and published statement setting out how it believes people with learning difficulties should be cared for. There should also be evidence that this statement is kept under review. Such a shared vision can be actively developed in a locality by encouraging multidisciplinary and multiagency discussion involving the clients (where possible), their advocates (if any), carers and top management. Despite firm intentions to ask clients their opinions whenever possible, this remains difficult when so many people with profound handicap are unable to speak for themselves. Consulting parents is an excellent idea, but can present complications. Some parents tend to be more vocal than others, some may not be aware of all the possibilities or underestimate what could be possible, and others' main motivation may be to gain peace of mind as opposed to the best outcome for the client. A citizen advocate could be useful to ensure the client's voice is heard (see Chapter 4). Set against this is the argument that professional staff have no right to say that they know best (see Chapter 8 for further discussion on professional power).

Marketing literature talks about a process of matching product benefits with customer wants, which must be monitored constantly. A company must define the benefits it offers or problems it solves for customers.

☐ **Philosophy of service**

Clarity of purpose is synonymous with having a philosophy of care. A series of training workshops, visits to places of good practice, and reading documents setting out recommended practice will help to develop an agreed philosophy of care. It is essential that the philosophy of care has all the relevant parties' commitment. This 'ownership' provides the bedrock on which it is possible to build a total quality service. It enables all decisions to be measured against a constant target. Without this philosophy, the service develops and managers are operating in shifting sand, where the ground rules are frequently changing. To illustrate this point, the following are two basic principles adopted by one health authority:

1. The goal is to 'see mentally handicapped people in the mainstream of life living in ordinary houses in ordinary streets, with the same range of choices as any citizen and mixing as equals with other and mostly non-handicapped members of their own community' (Kings Fund 1980).

2. People with a mental handicap have the same value and human rights as anyone else and they should be supported by means which are valued by society. (Campaign for Mental Handicap 1985).

Experience has shown that such explicitly stated principles prove invaluable in subsequent decision making. Clearly stated principles enable planners and managers to detect and reject inferior compromises, because it can be seen whether a service development fails to fit within these guiding principles. A typical example from one health authority was the suggestion that the challenging behaviour unit should be moved from a domestic-scale house in a prime community location (where it operated beneficially to the clients as they were able to participate easily in community life) to an isolated institutional setting in a large Victorian psychiatric hospital. While the planners thought this a sensible move, care staff could cite the agreed principle that a service for people with challenging behaviour should deviate as little as possible from basic principles. The proposed move was therefore avoided. It should be pointed out that clearly stated principles not only allow poor ideas to be detected and rejected, but help to identify the good ideas and opportunities for service development, so that it is easier and quicker to gain the commitment and support for action.

□ Service principles

The principles of a service are based on developing clear ideas of current values. What is the current view of people with learning difficulties in society today, and what standards of care does society expect from good local services?

The Independent Development Council for people with mental handicap (1987) listed principles to which a local service should adhere. A good quality local service is one which:

- Values the client as a full citizen with rights and responsibilities, entitled to be consulted about his or her needs and to have a say about plans that are being made to meet those needs, no matter how severe his or her learning difficulty may appear at first sight.

- Aims to promote the independence and to develop the skills and activities of both clients and families.

- Aims to design, implement and evaluate a programme of help which is based on the unique needs of each individual.

- Aims to help the client use ordinary services and resources of the local community such as primary care, education, health, employment, housing, welfare and recreational services.

- Aims to meet special needs arising from disabilities by means of locally fully coordinated multidisciplinary specialist services developed by appropriately trained staff.

- Is easily accessible.

- Is delivered to the client's home school or place of employment.

- Is delivered regardless of age or severity of disability.

- Plans actively to discharge people from institutions.

- Is staffed by locally based small teams.

Philosophy of care depends greatly on current public opinion as to what constitutes good care. The concept of 'product life cycle' can be usefully borrowed from business marketing literature. Examples of service products in health care are care management and group homes. According to the product life cycle concept it is possible to work out for any service examined whether it is in the introduction, growth, maturing, saturation or decline phase of the life cycle. Figure 2.2 shows the position on the product life cycle of group homes, care management and locally based hospital units.

The position of various components of the local service on the product life cycle should be regularly reviewed to ensure that service development is keeping pace with market changes.

A second major area that needs to be considered is the effect of service delivery on the lives of the people served. O'Brien (1987) has identified five ways in which services affect people's lives (see Chapter 8 for a fuller discussion). The first of these is community presence, such as community integration, which refers to using the same facilities as the rest of the community, as opposed to segregated facilities. Another important factor is that of relationships (see Chapter 5); there is a need to create opportunities for people to form valued relationships with non-handicapped people in a variety of work, education and leisure activities (see Chapter 6 for further information on leisure activities). Enabling clients to make choices is an

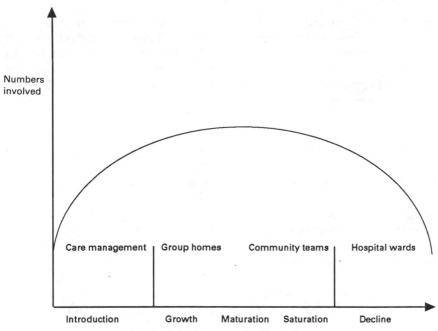

Figure 2.2 The service life cycle.

indicator of a quality service. A high quality service will give priority to facilitating clients to make choices which are available to everyone, regardless of the degree of learning difficulty. The protection of their human rights will also be a key issue. Ensuring clients receive a provision of assistance to become increasingly able to perform useful, meaningful and relevant activities, and to improve their competence, is also a fundamental aspect of quality care. Ensuring clients are respected as fellow human beings is the final service accomplishment. Services should set the example of treating people with learning difficulties as of similar status to other valued members of the community. A quality assurance tool is currently being developed in this country to assist services in measuring their success in meeting these accomplishments. This tool is called Equal IF, and it is based on Monitor (Cummings & Goldstone 1991). This is a quality assurance tool for use in residential services for adults with learning difficulties. It is based on well-known and accepted principles such as social role valorisation (see Chapters 1 and 4), ordinary life (see Chapter 1) as well as the five accomplishments (see Chapter 8).

☐ **Working practices**

A close look at working practices highlights the following issues. Working practices may be excellent, but available or accessible only to a small portion of potential users. This poses the question: 'How well do local services meet community need?'. Are they comprehensive in identifying and meeting the needs of all who would benefit and in providing the full range of necessary services? Are they appropriate, timely, accessible and coordinated around each individual user? Current good practice would recommend that some kind of individual programme planning system be included. There are various brands with various names, such as life planning and shared action planning, but they are all variations on a theme (see Chapter 8 for further discussion). The focus is on identifying individual needs, noting the strengths of the person and utilising these in writing out a positive action programme for meeting various objectives, based on the individual's needs. The client's participation in the process is recommended and only those professionals and contacts who know the client well should be involved. Such a system requires service commitment. Assessment of client skills and progress is an integral component of the evaluation of services. Plans written as specific objectives can be regularly monitored, and this presents one opportunity for quality assurance and for clinical audit. When plans are monitored, care should be taken to ensure that the plans address more than the meeting of the physical needs of clients. The plans of care should show a commitment to the five accomplishments for them to be regarded as being an acceptable indicator of quality.

Consideration of working practices would not be complete without the inclusion of issues to do with multidisciplinary team working. A team is a group of people who share common objectives and who need to work together to action them. Government policy has put pressure on Health Authorities and Local Authorities to develop community care. The common response has been to develop community mental handicap teams who are typically made up of a variety of professional disciplines, including social workers, community nurses, psychologists, psychiatrists and therapists, all of whom must discover improved ways to work collaboratively to deliver a quality service to the customer. This should involve ensuring that work is not duplicated by team members. As with other aspects of the service the community teams need to have a shared vision and philosophy for the service they offer. Team members should be fully aware of their roles and responsibilities within the team. The team should develop multidisciplinary team standards of practice to which all the team members adhere. The members of the team must be aware of their own limitations in meeting clients' needs. Indeed, the service quality of the community team depends on two factors. These are that team members know when to seek specialist skills and advice and they know which team member has this expertise.

■ Quality assurance

A current definition of quality assurance is a process which provides for the systematic evaluation of the quality of client care, i.e. an evaluation of the care provided. In addition to this, quality assurance should be able to demonstrate improvement of quality, where indicated by the results of evaluation. Client care is defined as all aspects of client care, including clinical care and all support and hotel services.

Quality assurance is essentially about (Quest for Health Care 1990):

- Developing a desired quality of service, which includes written standards of care.

- Measuring the care provided against these standards in order to detect those aspects of the service which are good as well as detecting the problem areas of the service.

Having identified the problem areas action is taken to solve the problems identified and this is followed up to ensure the problems have been solved.

A quality assurance procedure:

- Assesses the process and outcomes of care services.

- Applies agreed standards or indicators of quality.

- Considers resource utilisation if appropriate.

- Takes into account the view of the clients or the public.

- Focuses on problems shown to be affecting the quality of care.

- Identifies action required to solve problems.

- Follows up to determine if the action taken actually improved care.

To implement a quality assurance programme it is necessary to:

- Obtain agreement and commitment to the programme from all levels of staff.

- Have a system of collecting data which provides an objective measurement of actual practices against standards (Quest for Health Care 1990).

Johnson (1990) describes a simple but effective system for developing aims against which to measure performance. Using O'Brien's accomplishments as headings, examples of what staff think clients should be able to expect from a good service are elicited. An example of this is that, under the heading of relationships, an item could be 'being helped to send someone you like a birthday card'. A full list is elicited over a period of time. Staff are then asked to sort the list into categories, and those items which fall into the category of what happens now and can be observed and measured, and those which could happen in the near future if minor obstacles were removed, are put into a hat and six drawn out for consideration to decide the best method to audit these items. Monitoring methods were then worked out and implemented. Periodically, different items would be audited.

☐ **Customer views**

Customer feedback is a powerful evaluative tool. Many businesses use customer questionnaires to gain feedback on the service they offer. This approach is also being used in the health service. Parents of short-term care users (and users themselves) can fill in a questionnaire giving opinions on subjects such as arrangements on arriving at the unit, communication during the stay, conditions during the stay, arrangements for collecting relatives, perceptions of whether their relative enjoyed the stay, ratings of care received, comments of whether the service will be used again, and (last but not least) an open invitation to comment. However, care must be taken when analysing these data, as it is not uncommon for people to feel unable to criticise the service if they are aware that suitable alternatives do not exist. In addition to this, they may feel that if they are critical of the service this will result in their relative being penalised in some way by service providers or they may be concerned that they might be labelled 'trouble-makers'.

■ **Standard setting**

To generate standards it is necessary to get information about the resources available (structure), how they are used (process) and the eventual effects (outcomes). Thus, the outcome is the client's condition and feelings after receiving care. A standard is the point of reference. It can be seen to be a level of performance which is unacceptable, acceptable, excellent or opti-mum, and is related to criteria which can be used to determine success. Using the framework of structure, process, outcome and minimum/ maximum, levels of standards can be set which are observable measurable and achievable. Table 2.1 indicates a standard set in this way.

It is important to consider who should set standards. Standards need to be derived from a consensus of professional thinking and are therefore a multidisciplinary concern. It is initially possible to get each profession to state its own standards. These standards are then discussed and agreed by the multidisciplinary team. This approach ensures that there is a team standard of which every profession is aware and in agreement, and thus a holistic approach to care is taken. It is necessary to specify the areas for which each profession is responsible and for there to be an agreed philos-ophy of care which incorporates the profession's current values. People with learning difficulties and their advocates should be fully involved in setting

Table 2.1 Defining a standard

Topic	Freedom of choice
Care group	Learning difficulty
Standard statement	Each client chooses what he/she wants to do from the available activities
Monitoring method	Observation and recording

Structure	Process	Outcome
Wide range of activities available	Staff provide a variety of activities	Each client chooses what he or she wants to do from the available activities
Adequate space to enable different activities to occur	Staff enable clients to participate in a number of activities	Each client participates in the activity chosen
Programme of activities available	Staff assess clients' likes and dislikes	The client enjoys the chosen activity
1:2 staffing ratio	Staff adapt activities to suit clients' abilities	The client experiences a wide range of activity
	Staff assess clients' skills and needs in relation to activity	The clients' skill level increases

standards. Standards are set at the level of individual client outcome (life planning, shared action planning or individual programme planning systems can facilitate this – see Chapter 8 for further discussions) for residential or day services as individual units. They can also be set at care group level, district level and regional level. Each set of standards should be compatible with those set by the level above and below.

The following is an example of a standard set at care group level:

Each service user will have the opportunity to express their wishes and to plan goals by influencing decisions which shape their lives.

At ward/house level this statement would be that each client who uses the service participates in developing and evaluating their care plan. A district level standard might aim to determine service quality by stating that all action contained within the care plans adheres to nursing policies and procedures and that every practitioner has access to the policy and procedure documents. A regional level standard might state that all practioners and carers have available to them and implement current written standards of practice for all major aspects of care, and current written policies and procedures which reflect this standard (Wessex RHA 1990a). Thus standards at various level should be complementary and should fit together logically.

Standards can be set in those areas of practice which are giving cause for concern. This will enable a problem solving approach to be utilised to address those issues, whilst ensuring that the standards are regularly monitored and progress towards achievement noted. Standards should also be set in relation to the following areas:

- Values and objectives.
- Care practices.
- Policies and procedures.
- Personal planning.
- Education and training.
- Environment.
- Catering.

Writing standards in these areas will ensure that the environment in which people live and the standard of meals provided are also subject to the same rigorous monitoring as other aspects of the service. Including a standard in relation to staff education and training will ensure that quality staff with appropriate skills are available to the clients. This standard will also indicate to staff that they are also valued, and as such may improve their level of motivation.

■ Audit

One of the King's Fund quality project team (Brooks & Pitt 1990) is developing a national system of organisational audit based on the accreditation of services. So far, only acute hospitals have been involved, but the team is about to consider the needs of community care. The organisational audit system used is based on the Australian system of accreditation, and involves a hospital carrying out a self assessment against national standards, working out an action plan from this and then submitting to a visit from a survey team. It is stressed that there can be no guarantee that the service provided will be a quality one, but it does help to ensure that an accredited service has in place all the mechanics of management to ensure that quality is possible. Auditing a service involves some kind of measurement of service provision. This is usually carried out by the observation method. In an attempt to ensure that the audit is objective, the observation is usually carried out by someone external to the care group. It can be seen that this can conflict with the service philosophy. Where clients live in their own homes the issue of whether we have the right of access to monitor the care provided must be addressed. The dangers of not auditing the service outweigh the strict adherence to service philosophy. If an audit is not conducted, poor care will not be detected and clients may continue to receive a quality of care which at best is unacceptable and at worst may be harmful. However, audit must be carried out with sensitivity and preferably with the client's or their advocate's agreement. If the client has an advocate then this may be the most suitable person to conduct the audit, as they want to ensure their 'friend' receives the best possible care.

■ Quality employer

Yet another facet of the quality assurance debate is to do with the organisation attempting to become a quality employer by working out a human resource strategy (Wessex RHA 1990b). Aspects which need to be addressed in any human resource strategy are in relation to ensuring that the correct skill mix of staff is available to deliver a quality service. Staff development and individual performance reviews for staff are essential to ensure that the right people with the right level of skills are deployed effectively within the organisation. This means that staff must have access to and be encouraged to participate in training opportunities in order to develop the necessary skills to provide the services at the level required. Other chapters in this book indicate some areas where staff training is important and Chapter 11 focuses specifically on education and training issues. It is essential that a quality employer has a good communication strategy. Without this, staff will be unclear about the philosophy of the employer and will be unsure if they are meeting the employer's current and future objectives. A communication strategy should ensure that staff understand and are committed to the organisational changes which may occur.

■ Conclusion

It can be seen that quality can be viewed from many perspectives and has many elements. The issues which need addressing are varied and complex. They require time and effort from people at every level of the organisation in order to determine what constitutes a quality service for their organisation within the allocated resources. It is worth reiterating that when implementing quality measures the expectation is that staff provide the best quality of care they can within the resources available to them. Thus quality is of central importance because it alone can assure effective service delivery. Most important of all, it puts the focus on the client and client outcomes and measures performance.

■ References

Brooks, T. & Pitt, C. (1990). *Organisational audit (Accreditation for an acute hospital)*. King Edward's Hospital Fund for London.

Campaign for Mental Handicap (1985). *The principle of normalisation*. CMH Publications, London.

Cummings, M. & Goldstone, L. (1991). *Equal IF Evaluating quality using assessment of lifestyles – Individuals first. A quality assurance package for use in residential services for adults who have a learning difficulty*. Gale Centre Publications, London.

Department of Health (1990a). *The National Health Service and Community Care Act 1990*. HMSO, London.

Department of Health (1990b). *Caring for people*. HMSO, London.

Independent Development Council (1987). *Pursing Quality*. Independent Development Council, London.

Johnson, D. (1990). Steps to a better service. *Health Care Journal*, June.

King's Fund (1980). *An ordinary life*. King Edward's Hospital Fund for London.

O'Brien, J. (1987). *A guide to personal future planning*. Responsive Systems Associates, Georgia USA.

Quest for Health Care (1990). *Manual for medical audit assistants*. Healthcare Quality Quest, Romsey.

Wessex RHA (1990a). *Guidelines for development of standards for nursing services providing care for people with a mental handicap in the Wessex region*. Wessex RHA, Winchester.

Wessex RHA (1990b). *Putting people first*. Wessex RHA, Winchester.

Wieck, C., Nelson, J., Reedstrom, C., Starr, J. & Stone, N. (1989). *Quality assurance resources*. Association for Retarded Citizens, Texas USA.

Chapter 3

Planning and managing change

Patricia Brigden

■ Introduction

Change is an unavoidable fact of life. The change process is dynamic and can have complex ramifications within an organisation. It is important to recognise the signs that change is needed and then to be able to manage the process. In order to control the process, a carefully designed strategy needs to be implemented systematically and not in an *ad hoc* manner. Everyone should be involved, including clients. Clients are rarely remembered when planning changes and yet they are always the most affected. If an advocacy system is established (see Chapter 4), then it should be possible to get clients' views fed into the process. Change becomes necessary either because of external or internal pressures. Currently the overriding factors pressing for change are external: the National Health Service reforms and the focus on community care covered by the National Health Service and Community Care Act 1990. It is well known that people dislike change and therefore tend to resist it. The reasons for this will be covered later in this chapter.

This chapter will explore a number of change management strategies which could prove useful. The current changes in the National Health Service will be explored in relation to the need to be knowledgeable about change strategies. However, the strategies described can be used when making any kind of changes; that is, they work for limited changes to do with individuals as well as for major changes at service level.

■ Context

The pace of change at the present time is rapid. The National Health Service and Community Care Act (Department of Health 1990) proposes such a range and depth of change that it will be some time before the government vision of what the finalised service should look like becomes fully evident.

Already the concept of provider units separated from a purchasing function is a familiar one. District Health Authorities have become purchasers. This will enable District Health Authorities as purchasers to contract with provider units of their choice in the internal market. Thus there will be cross-boundary flows. The money will follow the individual in need of care. Some provider units have already become self-governing trusts. The remainder are aiming for Trust status in the third wave, i.e. by April 1993.

It seems likely that the future character of the service will be multi-agency; that purchasers will not be looking for traditional placements; and that purchasers will be aiming to provide only that service/care which is required.

The mechanism on which the new National Health Service depends is a contracting system within cash limits. Under the annual agreement any provider unit receives a fixed amount of cash at the start of the year from its purchaser(s) in return for agreeing to supply specified services to specified people. It will become increasingly important for the provider units to establish in advance the likely purchasing patterns and to build up a number of different purchasers to assist their chances of staying in business.

Thus, proactive external appraisal enabling accurate forecasting is the best chance there is of planning sensibly for the effects of changes in the volume of service required. Contingency planning for services for people with learning difficulties will be essential. If a very small service suddenly has to double the staff support for one individual and this factor has not been built into the contract, the effect on the financial picture could be drastic. There are already accounts of provider units experiencing financial difficulties. In one example the purchaser moved the clients, while in a second example the 'private' organisation had over-mortgaged itself.

In addition to the changes outlined above, the full implementation of community care is anticipated in the near future. Social services are now the lead agency for services for people with a learning difficulty. As such they will be expected to take responsibility for assessing client needs and for purchasing suitable tailored individual packages of care. Until recently, clients discharged from Health Service care were able to claim enhanced benefits. This situation encouraged the setting up of a growing number of housing consortium projects, where health, social services and voluntary agencies are collaborating with housing associations, to set up a range of sheltered residential options where discharged clients can live in the community supported by the degree of staffing input that they need. The Government has now changed the benefit system so that discharged clients can no longer claim such favourable benefit allowances. This is currently causing housing consortia to search actively for other means of funding new services.

The market envisaged for clients with learning difficulties could become quite complex. Provider units could be run by the Department of Health, Social Services, the voluntary sector, the private sector or by a combination of these.

☐ **Product life cycle**

The rapidly changing context of service delivery resulting from the implementation of the government White Paper has been superimposed on whatever stage of evolution local services had reached. In Chapter 2 the concept of product life cycle was introduced. This concept has been adopted from business literature and applied to describing service models. It was explained that owing to current public opinion and current government guidance the national trend is for services to move away from old Victorian institutions (hospitals) which are thus contracting and closing down, and increasingly moving towards community care. Different people have different ideas as to what constitutes community care. It is defined here as 'an ordinary life, in an ordinary house in an ordinary street' (see Chapter 1), and is underpinned by the value base that a person with a learning difficulty is a person with rights who should be supported in ways that are valued by society. However, this view is not shared by everyone concerned with people with learning difficulties. Some people tend to see segregated villages as community care, and consider this a preferable model (more realistic, more practical, more affordable) to the fully integrated, dispersed model. Such views are still to be found among staff in institutions, and also among many parents who see villages as a home for life and thus perceive security and peace of mind as more likely outcomes than opting for the riskier dispersal/integration model. This model has also been endorsed by the junior Minister for Health (McMillan 1991). In contrast, currently the latest service model in the life cycle is care management. A recent advertisement for a Director of Learning Difficulty Service stated that the post-holder would have 'responsibility for a budget for the purchase of "packages of care" provided by the statutory, voluntary and independent sectors for over 70 people'.

It can be seen that in any situation, the service model will reflect a stage in evolution which can be described. This is Position A. Position B would be a description of what the service should ideally look like in the full knowledge of excellent quality practices elsewhere. The task is to move from A to B as rapidly as possible, taking into account cultural peculiarities, views and needs of people with learning difficulties, staff and parent attitudes and availability of resources.

■ The manager as change agent

The working environment is changing, but this merely emphasises the need for skills and knowledge in planning and implementing change. Quite simply, this chapter is about *how* to implement changes of all types successfully, within organisations.

Managers must be able to recognise the role that other individuals and groups within the organisation have to play in the change process. They may be trying to introduce their own idea, or they may be responsible for implementing changes decided by others, possibly their superiors. In all cases it is essential to convince others that the proposed change is feasible and necessary, or it will not be successfully implemented. This is a process known as 'internal marketing'.

People perceive situations differently. Some see change as an opening or an opportunity, others see it as a threat to the familiar or established situation. People's perceptions are thus important. People are more likely to regard negatively change which is imposed on them than change over which they have some control. Organisational change may be precipitated by external forces or by pressure from within. Not every change that takes place results in operational reorganisation; it is well known that organisations tend to remain unchanged despite pressures. This leads to the concept of restraining forces as well as driving forces at work in an organisation. The concept of Force Field Analysis suggests that an organisation is held in balance by the interaction of two opposing sets of forces – those seeking to promote change (driving forces) and those attempting to maintain the status quo (restraining forces): see Figure 3.1.

The major difference between externally and internally driven change is degree of control. If change is driven externally the organisation is forced to react (reactive approach), but if change is internally generated it is better understood and should be controlled from inception to completion (the 'proactive' approach).

Staff response to change varies enormously. Those at the top, responsible for introducing change, may be enthusiastic and excited while many of the long-term employees may be apprehensive and afraid. Both long-term employees who remember the past and new employees who have not yet had time to establish credibility may find rapid change especially stressful. Personal response to change is more to do with feeling in control of one's own future than to do with whether change is internally or externally driven.

People may find themselves in a situation which needs to be changed. The problem is to decide how to go about making the change.

Alternatively there may be tensions caused by influences and pressures for change on a person's situation but no clear idea of the area or direction of the change that is needed. In this situation it is not yet possible to consider how to implement change.

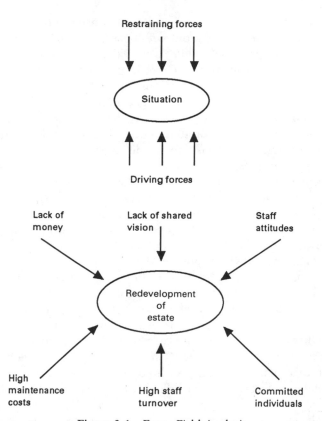

Figure 3.1 Force Field Analysis.

The second situation is both more complex and more difficult than the first. Problems range from comparatively easy ones, where it is known what needs to be done and concern centres on how best to effect change (i.e. on methodology) to difficult ones where it seems impossible to identify where one wants to get (the desired objective). Intractable problems tend to be the latter kind!

The Open University (1987) describes a problem situation which is unsolvable in the daily routine as a 'mess'. A 'mess' is a situation where there is no clarity about the type of change needed, what it will involve, who will be affected and what will be achieved. To make a problem manageable it has to be defined in a way that enables it to be extracted from its background. If this is successfully achieved it is known who is involved and what needs to be done, when and by whom to solve the problem. Thus the priorities become clear. In contrast everything about a 'mess' is uncertain. The perception of the problem keeps changing, so it is impossible to see what possible solutions there might be. The full implications are not known.

☐   **Taking account of individual differences**

People's perceptions of problems vary, and consequently it can never be assumed that problem resolution will be easy. Without other people's agreement to the proposed solution it will not work. It is possible to demonstrate that individual differences in personal and work experiences result in sufficiently different perceptions that conflict over goals, directions and strategy become inevitable. One type of cultural clash might be a manager's view and a union representative's view over the same strike situation.

What people are willing or able to do about problems is often affected by role constraints. Any position in an organisation has expectations attached to it and the post-holder will be acutely aware of these. Thus a psychologist in one organisation may hold a leading role in determining how the service develops and is delivered, while a psychologist in an apparently similar organisation may be actively discouraged to think beyond face to face contact with clients. The role is the resulting pattern of behaviour permitted by the expectations of others. These expectations set limits to what any individual post-holder can do.

To free up and enable an organisation to effect change it is useful to examine the influences on the individual positions in the organisation. Who has the power to change and who does not? Are those who are able to change the structure and systems the people who need to have that power? It may be that the people who have the skills and ability to affect change are rendered impotent by the system. Change management involves altering systems rather than changing post-holders. This is because a new post-holder will be subject to the same influences and is likely to behave similarly in the role.

Staff have had different experiences of education, work and background. These individual differences result in varying perspectives about what problems are and how they can be dealt with. For example, at a training event the participants were asked how to defuse a potential riot. A trainee chaplain suggested offering tea and biscuits, while a farm hand suggested letting a bull loose.

These perspectives must be borne in mind when attempting to influence somebody. It is important to try to find out why individuals think the way they do. This leads to common ground, which enables talking to start. Obtaining a shared perspective is crucial to problem solving. What one has to avoid is prematurely offering obvious solutions which others dismiss because of their differing cultural backgrounds.

Problem solving involves:

● describing and clarifying the nature of the problem.

● obtaining information.

- obtaining cooperation from others.

- negotiating an agreement.

- obtaining commitment to an agreed action plan.

Working with others is very important. Firstly, talking to the person may introduce some new ideas. Secondly, you will be 'perceived' to be working collaboratively. As has been said already, without cooperation the solution will not happen.

☐ Getting started

As situations of change are usually very complex and involve large numbers of interacting factors, it can be helpful to learn simple diagramming techniques and conventions. The following are examples of diagrams to show how helpful they can be in clarifying the picture (Figures 3.2 and 3.3). They represent a sample of a large number of types of diagramming techniques available (Open University 1987).

☐ Management of DHA's service for people with learning difficulties

Figure 3.4 is an example of a systems map to show who the core team and the wider team consist of and the interfaces involved. This systems map indicates where services for people with learning difficulties fit within the management structure for a Health Authority. Figure 3.5 indicates the environmental influences on the service for people with learning difficulties, and Figure 3.6 indicates some factors which may be involved in generating change in these services. Services can respond to these pressures to change in a variety of ways (See Figure 3.7).

☐ Methodology

There are a number of systems approaches available for managing change. Some methods originate from engineering and concentrate primarily on 'objects', so are known as 'hard' methods. Others concentrate on people in organisations, and, because this introduces a 'messy' element, are known as 'soft' methods. Any systems approach to change can be described as 'harder' or 'softer' depending on whether its emphasis is more on 'objects' or more on 'people'. In a care service soft approaches are the method of choice.

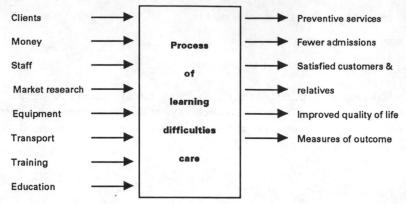

Figure 3.2 Input–output model of service to show required outcomes for people with learning difficulties.

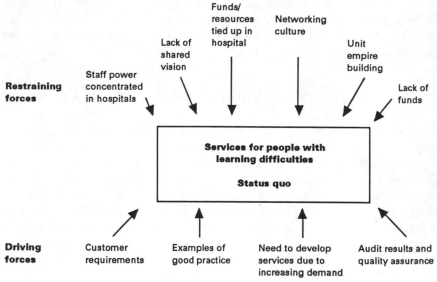

Figure 3.3 Force Field Analysis showing how the status quo is maintained.

Two particularly useful methods are discussed here (Open University 1987): systems intervention strategy and organisational development. The former is 'harder' than organisational development, but is still process orientated, a feature of 'soft' methods. Organisational development concentrates on people and their setting. Systems intervention strategy involves three stages:

Stage 1 Description of problem
Hypothesis adopted
Objectives and measures worked out

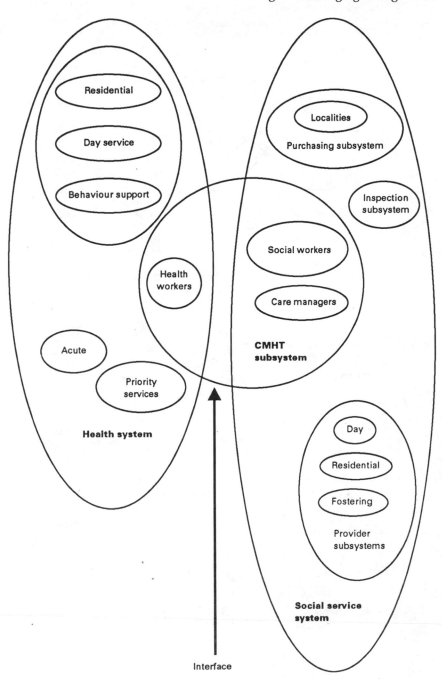

Figure 3.4 Systems map for the core team and the wider team in a District Health Authority.

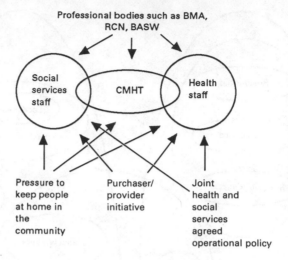

Figure 3.5 Environmental influences on the service provided.

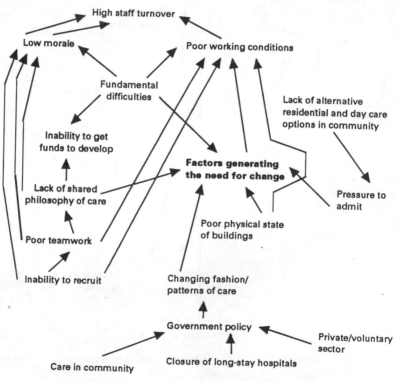

Figure 3.6 Factors involved in generating change.

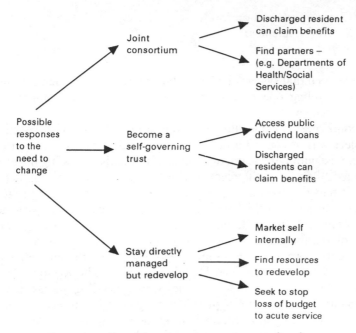

Figure 3.7 Possible responses to pressures for change.

Stage 2 Change options: identified
                                       compared
                                       selection of best

Stage 3 Options compared to preset criteria
Implementation
Evaluation

Throughout, the project manager must keep checking with the problem owner(s) to make sure that he or she is getting it right.

The stages are broken down into steps:

Stage 1 Description of problem
    Step 1 find a way in and use systems diagramming to aid definition process
    Step 2 identify objectives and constraints
    Step 3 specify how achievement of objective is to be recognised

Stage 2 Change options
    Step 1 generate options by brainstorming
    Step 2 for each option work out who does what, when, where and how

Stage 3 Choose preferred option
  Step 1 implement
  Step 2 monitor

It can be seen that systems intervention strategy is a thorough, systematic process enabling one to take an organised and logical approach to change management.

The following example illustrates the approach in action. A clinical audit project was attempted and failed on a hospital ward. Differences of opinion existed within the team, one influential member insisting the project be continued, the rest of the team insisting it could not. The conflict was such that it had the potential to seriously jeopardise operational practice. There was a generally held belief that personality clashes between team members were the cause of failure. A new project manager was given the task of resolving the problem and implementing an audit project.

The situation was further complicated by the need to complete a contract as agreed with the Regional Health Authority. The Regional Health Authority had backed the project and they were providing the assistance of a management consultant. It was therefore a high profile project, and failure would be embarrassing for a number of senior managers.

The scenario as described is a typical 'mess'. An apparently straightforward task of implementing a simple audit project had turned out to be more complex than anticipated. It was unclear what the problem was, and who and how many people were involved. The implications of the proposals were greater than was originally supposed and it was no longer clear what should be done and by when results could be achieved.

Initial moves involved attempts to diagnose what was occurring. To gain entry to the problem some systems diagramming was carried out (as in Figure 3.4) to work out who the core team were and who the wider team were. A semi-structured interview was constructed and everyone identified during the systems diagramming was interviewed. Information obtained from the interviews was used to identify objectives and constraints. The main issues identified were a need for multidisciplinary coordination, shared vision and agreed working practices (an operational policy). It could be seen that if the team was meeting regularly, had discussed and agreed a philosophy document (for shared vision), and had worked out an operational policy the objectives would be met.

To commence the work an away-day was held for the wider team. The day consisted of group work involving techniques such as brainstorming to generate a range of ideas as to how to implement the audit. At the end of this day the project manager had been given approval by the group to prepare the preferred option in detail.

One of the constraints identified was lack of time for the team to meet, and it was agreed that it would be possible to meet for one hour per month over a six-month period to achieve the objectives. This monthly meeting was used to discuss draft papers on a range of topics which included philosophy and aspects of a ward operational policy. Prior to implementing and evaluating this plan the project manager discussed the proposals with the problem owners. Before the end of the six month time-scale, working practices had been agreed to the degree that staff volunteered themselves as ready and able to participate in a repeat of the audit project. This time it was successfully implemented.

These types of problem could be dealt with in another way.

If one imagines oneself with a camera looking at a scene then it will be realised that decisions have to be made about the degree of detail to include in the picture. Either the camera can focus on close-up detail or it can stand back using a wide-angled lens to get a broader but less detailed view. What is it you are really interested in knowing? Figure 3.6 shows the factors generating a need for change in a service for people with a learning difficulty. Figure 3.7 lists options for change.

A strategy is a plan which allows the change process to be managed, but is flexible enough to cater for issues raised by those affected. All stakeholders need to be involved and to participate. Stakeholders are those people likely to be affected by the change. It is important to give the message that people matter, so making consultation plans alone can help to make this point. However, a proper process of consultation ensures that people know what is going on. The timing of involving people is critically important. If it is left too late consultation tends not to have the required effect. This timing factor is called the window of opportunity. Bar charts and critical path analysis are used to plan transition from position A to position B, where position A is the current situation and position B is the desired future position.

Sometimes the change strategy envisages total change, but this is risky. Occasionally change strategy involves pilot studies (which spread if successful), or parallel training (where old systems run alongside new systems). This latter strategy is time-consuming and involves duplication. Different strategies suit different situations. Pilot studies tend to be popular.

☐ **The change process**

Pugh (1978) analyses the change process by looking at what is going on in four major areas.

1. Adequacy of planning (How well were people persuaded? Did they have enough time to assimilate the information?)

2. Account taken of occupational and political impact

3. Account taken of reasoned discussion

4. Appropriateness of starting point and methods

Pugh's principles can be used to analyse why a carefully thought out joint health/social services strategy in one Health Authority was unsuccessful in achieving change. Firstly, the planning, though careful, was academic rather than practical in nature. They were only superficially getting others 'on board'. As soon as the political situation changed these doubtful supporters of change ceased to support it at all. A close look at why these individuals were indifferent and apathetic about the proposed change revealed that the likely occupational impact was perceived to be too great a price to pay if it could be avoided. Change is inevitably resented by some people.

Huse (1975) lists several factors which decrease resistance to change:

1. Needs, attitudes and beliefs of 'stakeholders' to be considered (what are the personal benefits for them?)

2. Stakeholders to have adequate prestige, power and influence

3. Stakeholders to share vision of need for change

4. The group must be cohesive

5. The leader must be involved

6. Communication channels must be opened and information must be shared

7. Feedback on results must be supplied

Huse's factors are features of examples of successful change.

The following is an example where all Huse's elements for decreasing resistance were effectively utilised. A residential unit was closed down by moving residents into several group homes. It was then re-opened for fewer people with the same staffing establishment, but with the brief to care for people with challenging behaviour. In this situation all staff were involved and consulted from the beginning. The manager interviewed every member of staff personally, explained the reasons for change and elicited support for it. The practical ramifications were outlined, including listing all likely employment options, and staff were invited to state their preferences for jobs in the proposed new service. As far as possible, people were fitted into jobs of their first and second choice. Open meetings were held at regular intervals to share factual information, and suggestions were welcomed. Staff also participated actively in the process of deciding which resident went where, and in the furnishing and equipping of the new homes.

The organisational development process (Albrecht 1983) is an explicit strategy for initiating change and managing the process. It is a cyclical set of sequential stages which recurs:

1. Look at the environment

2. What are the problems and the opportunities?

3. Educate to obtain understanding of implications for the organisation

4. Get people involved in the project (take into account perceived needs of participants)

5. Identify objectives for change

6. Change/development activities

7. Evaluate and reinforce change
   (Repeat from Step 1)

The following is an example.

1. *Environmental change*   Introduction of purchasers and providers.

2. *Identification of implications*   Health and Social Services may decide to organise themselves differently, for example Health horizontally and Social Services vertically. This will make working together very difficult.

3. *Education*   Discussion among senior managers for all agencies involved at relevant meetings, particularly joint forums between Health and Social Services.

4. *Involvement*   There has been little opportunity for those likely to be affected to join in these discussions. Decisions are being made at the top, so there is little chance of influencing events for those who will have to carry out new working practices.

5. *Targets for change*   Change levels at which decisions are made.

6. *Activities*   Experimental devolution of decision making.

7. *Evaluation*   Conference to review joint working arrangements.

   Any manager who wants to initiate change has a number of organisational development strategies to choose from. When attempting the diagnosis of the organisational development process, Pugh's matrix (1978) (see Figure 3.8) is helpful. It has two dimensions: level and type of intervention. Level can be 'individual', 'group', 'intergroup' or 'organisation'. This represents where change is needed. By types of intervention Pugh means whether it is 'behaviour', 'structure/systems' or 'context' that need to be the focus of change.
   When analysing an organisation one sees presenting symptoms such as reluctance to consider change; tasks too hard or too easy; mismatch between recognition and objectives; leader not respected; conflict; lack of awareness of environmental changes; and many more. Each symptom is indicative of problems at one of the levels. Thus lack of awareness of environmental changes points to problems at the organisational level; conflict suggests problems at an intergroup level; lack of respect for the leader

Level

	Individual	Group	Intergroup	Organisation
Behaviour				
Structure systems				
Context				

Type of intervention

Figure 3.8   Pugh's matrix.

suggests problems at a group level; and a mismatch between recognition and objectives a problem at an individual level.

Once the level of the problem has been identified, the type of intervention required must be identified. This is done by thinking about what happens now (behaviour), what system(s) are required (structure), and what setting is required (the context).

Current behaviours can be tackled directly without intervening into systems of settings. Intervention can be seen as overcoming difficulties in the effective and efficient workings of the current system. An example would be when team-building exercises are used to facilitate the effectiveness and efficiency of the multidisciplinary team, resulting in improved functioning, improved morale and a better standard of care.

This intervention, however, might not be sufficient in itself. Occasionally, regardless of the improvement in the group atmosphere and leadership style, the team still does not perform. This may be because the team is unclear as to what is required of it. Important information is missing and tasks are poorly allocated to group members, and in this case attention needs to be given to reorganising the system, i.e. working on structure, systems, information flow and job design. If this degree of intervention is still insufficient, the problem may be in the contextual setting (such as physical distance, market pressures, poor promotion procedures). Change strategy in these areas involves expensive and time-consuming use of resources and is therefore a last resort.

According to Pugh (1978), at the individual level change strategies for behaviour could be counselling, role analysis and career planning; at the structure level they could be job restructuring, job enrichment and management by objectives; at the context level they could be, for example, person-nel changes or improved training and education.

At the group level, change strategies for behaviour could be process consultation and team building; at the structure level they could be rede-signing work relationships or forming autonomous working groups; at the context level they could be layout or group composition. At the inter-group level, change strategies could be inter-group confrontation (with a third party as consultant) and role negotiation; at the structure level they could be redefining responsibilities, changing reporting relationships, improving coordination and liaison mechanisms. At the context level, change strategies could be reducing distance or attachments. At the organisational level, change strategies for behaviour could be survey feedback; at the structure level a change strategy could be to change the structure; at the context level it could be a change of location or at the cultural level it could be the use of organisational development technique.

An example at this stage may help to clarify how Pugh's (1978) organi-sational development matrix can be used. A psychologist, on moving to a new job, discovered that in an apparently well-organised, smooth-running service, there was nevertheless every opportunity to come into conflict with some of the nursing staff. There was little evidence of therapists, who took a back-seat role. It seemed the less evident they were the more they were esteemed by users. The consultant was busy and overstretched and kept out of things as far as possible. There was evidence of unresolved feelings to do with prejudice and stereotypes of the different professional roles. Also, no one seemed to have confronted the differences in priorities between different professional groups in trying to achieve a good level of service delivery.

Clearly the problem was at an inter-group level and was largely related to what was happening at the time (behaviour). Recommended strategies were role negotiation or inter-group confrontation (with a third party as consultant). In this example there was also a lack of integrated task perspec-tive. This is an inter-group level problem, but it requires structural change. Recommended strategies would be redefining responsibilities, changing re-porting relationships and improving coordination and liaison mechanisms.

☐ **Success factors**

For a change strategy to succeed it is important to consider who needs to change, and how; to think it through; to get discussion going; to consider how to hear of objections and how to deal with them; to obtain and use the views of practitioners; and to monitor and reinforce change (Pugh 1978). To effect change in an organisation it is necessary to get people to think and believe in the need for it. Carnall (1990) lists ways to achieve this: job rotation; education/training; communication; creation of a climate which supports experiment and risk-taking; participation; ensuring innovation appears on all agendas; project groups; and identification and use of product champions. Product champions are committed enthusiasts whose extensive experience and dedication give them power-based knowledge. A product champion can be a charismatic leader and a powerful supporter for a cause if empowered by the system.

Plant (1987) outlines a number of practical ideas for vision-building work with groups of staff.

Kotter and Schlesinger (1979) believe the choice of change method must match the requirements of staff, resources available and time-scale. Methods range from training through participation, facilitation, negotiation, manipulation and coercion. The former methods are people-orientated and more likely to achieve success with the lasting support of the stakeholders. The latter methods may be appropriate for example in crisis situations.

Alexander (1985) describes successful change as the result of five stages: communication; a good idea; obtaining commitment and involvement; resources; and an implementation plan.

Slatter (1984) describes an eight-stage recovery strategy for ailing business. When the new manager arrives, he or she gains control; establishes credibility; assesses existing managers and replaces if necessary; evaluates the business; plans action; implements change; motivates management and employees; and installs or improves budgetary systems.

□ Coping with change

Changes which have a significant impact on the work that people do have an impact on their self-esteem (Kirkpatrick 1985). Linked to this is an impact on performance.

There is a learning curve effect (see Figure 3.9) as people build performance through learning about new systems and so on. Carnall (1990) describes a coping cycle (Figure 3.10).

Because stress is an outcome of change, careful thought needs to be given to pacing change so that no one is overfaced.

□ Helping clients change

Last, but not least, it should not be forgotten that one of the primary functions of staff working with people with learning difficulties is to facilitate changes either in the client's behaviour and/or skill level, or in his or her immediate environment. Little will be said here about skills-building techniques or behaviour therapy as these subjects have been extensively covered elsewhere. Suffice it to say that analytical tools that can be applied to organisations can often be adapted to thinking about the circumstances of

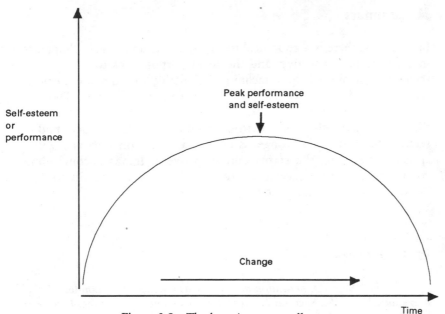

Figure 3.9 The learning curve effect.

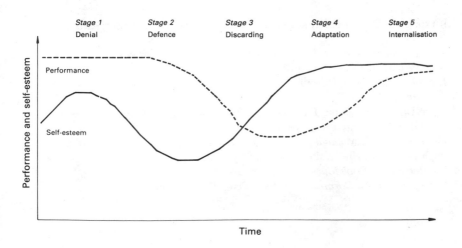

Figure 3.10 The coping cycle.

an individual, and can add an extra dimension to assessment, treatment and training for clients.

■ Summary

In summary, there is a good deal to say about 'change'. This chapter is not intended to be exhaustive, and the main purpose was to take the reader through some of the helpful techniques available and to relate them to care services, especially services for people with learning difficulties. This subject, always important, has never been so essential as it is now. The reason for this is the rapidly changing environmental context that services find themselves in at present. No longer is change an occasional activity with long spells of managing the status quo in between. It has become almost a continuous activity as services evolve to survive (and hopefully to flourish) in the new world of the 1990s.

■ References

Albrecht, K. (1983). *Organisation development*. Prentice-Hall, London.
Alexander, L. (1985). Successfully implementing strategic decisions. *Long Range Planning* **18** (3), 91–7.
Carnall, C. (1990). *Managing change in organisations*. Prentice-Hall, London.
Department of Health (1990). *NHS and Community Care Act 1990*. HMSO, London.
Huse, E. (1975). *Organisation development and change*. West Publishing Co., London.
Kirkpatrick, D. (1985). *How to manage change effectively*. Jossey Bass, New York.
Kotter, J. & Schlesinger, L. (1979). Choosing strategies for change. *Harvard Business Review* Mar/April.
McMillan, I. (1991). Dorrell pledges RNMHs will not be discarded. *Nursing Times* **87** (27), 7.
Open University Course Team (1987). *P679 Planning and managing change*. Open University Press, Milton Keynes.
Plant, R. (1987). *Managing change and making it stick*. Fontana, London.
Pugh D. (1978). Undertaking and managing organisational change. *London Business School Journal* **3** (2), 29–34.
Slatter, S. (1984). *Corporate strategy*. Penguin, Harmondsworth.

Chapter 4

Advocacy

Jo Young

■ Introduction

Various advocacy movements for people with learning difficulties have been developed in Britain over the last twenty years. The 1960s and 1970s were an unparalleled time of social unrest in the United Kingdom and America. They created a climate of self-determination, self-direction, assertion of specific interests and an active announcement of the need for the rights to citizenship to be acknowledged (Rhoades *et al*. 1986). The slogan 'power to the people' emerged as a true reflection of the energy of this era. For many minority groups, including people with learning difficulties, an outcry was made for social reform.

This period of advocacy brought about dramatic change. A brief history of events, which will provide an overview of how these changes developed into today's advocacy, will be described. The two most recognised types of advocacy, which are self-advocacy and citizen advocacy, will be discussed. In addition, new approaches to the practice of services that may have resulted from the influences of the advocacy movement will be outlined.

■ History

The historical legacy of terms such as of 'feeble-minded', 'idiot' or 'lunatic' remains embodied in many assumptions made about people with a learning difficulty (Sang & O'Brien 1984). In the 1960s these assumptions began to be challenged and the concept of advocacy began to emerge. The roots of advocacy are found in Sweden and America. In Sweden there was a network of leisure facilities for people with learning difficulties and it was proposed that a consultative body be established. To enable people to participate in this, courses on committee work and voting were arranged for people with learning difficulties. Rapid growth of self-advocacy began, and the network of clubs had a network of user representatives who met to discuss issues and share experiences. Regional conferences provided the foundation for the first national self-advocacy conference, which occurred in 1968 (Williams & Shoultz 1982). A three-day conference and broadcasting in 1970 attracted the rest of the world, planting the idea of advocacy in America and Britain (Sines 1988; Williams & Shoultz 1982). Policy documents and legislation also had traces of acknowledgement of people's rights to citizenship. In Britain, the White Paper Better Services for the Mentally Handicapped (DHSS 1971), indicated that there were a large number of isolated residents in 'care' and pointed out the contribution that could be made by using private citizens to mitigate this loneliness. There was emphasis on the value this type of informal voluntary befriending scheme would have. In December 1971 the United Nations Declaration of Rights of Mentally Retarded Persons was adopted (United Nations 1971). This embodied the principles of equality, integration, individualised habilitation, periodic review and natural justice (Sang & O'Brien 1984).

Shearer, stimulated by the national conference, returned to Britain and founded the Campaign for People with a Mental Handicap (Shearer 1986), and in 1972 held the first self-advocacy conference in Britain. The views of the 22 people with learning difficulties that attended that day were subsequently published (Sines 1988). American representatives from Oregon, excited by the Swedish conference, formalised the self-advocacy movement by creating People First, an organisation run by people with learning difficulties. Their first conference was in 1973 and soon after this People First became an international organisation with a British branch being established in London in 1984 (Booth 1990). The organisation compaigned for equal rights, equal responsibilities and equal opportunities, as they were equal people and wanted to be seen as people first. During the Year of the Disabled in 1981, a pilot project was established to provide citizen advocates for people living in three different hospitals. This project was to be named 'Advocacy Alliance' (Sines 1988; Sang & O'Brien 1984). In 1976 a similar scheme in a Sheffield hospital had successfully created a local citizen's advice bureau for the residents. A similar venture occurred in 1982 at Tooting Hill hospital.

Self-advocacy and citizen advocacy have tended to be developed simultaneously. There was a noticeable growth of groups and projects in the 1980s and a survey conducted in 1980 and repeated in 1986 provided evidence of this (Dowson 1990a). In 1988 a popular newspaper suggested there had been an increase from 40 to 300 self-advocacy groups in Britain. The British People First movement found a temporary office from which to operate in 1989 and in 1990 moved to permanent accommodation which they share with Values into Action (the former CMH). The organisation is aware of over 100 People First groups in the United Kingdom (Booth 1990).

■ Self-advocacy

□ Definition

The most common translation of self-advocacy is 'speaking out for yourself'; however Wolfensberger (1972) distinguishes between discussion and self expression and those acts of self determination which assist in clarifying important issues. Williams & Shoultz (1982) take this point further, developing self-advocacy into a dynamic mode which includes action and achievement of goals established through speaking out. The definition described in Sang & O'Brien (1984) states that self-advocacy occurs when people with a disability assert their own rights, needs and concerns, and assume the duties of full citizenship. Rights with responsibilities is a succinct description (Booth 1990). These definitions are important, as advocacy may be a buzz-word (Dowson 1990a), but it is hardly everyday language in the United Kingdom. Adding the prefix 'self' makes it a term which has no meaning to people who are outside of the services. This jargon therefore, may cloak and confuse the activity, thus limiting the practical benefits (Downson 1990b).

As stated earlier, the self-advocacy movement has grown. The increased amount of research and experience dispelled the belief that people with learning difficulties depended solely on others and needed protection from the stresses of ordinary life (Booth 1990), proving their supposed inabilities to be absent (Sines 1988). The increase of skills-teaching enabled people with learning difficulties to improve their choices and to articulate their views more effectively. Self-advocacy groups have allowed people to practice this and gain experience as a consumer. The essence has been the grass roots development of small peer groups offering support and the opportunity to master self-advocacy skills (Sines 1988).

□ Labelling

One of the first points that people with learning difficulties addressed was the fact that they were seen as handicapped first and people second. In a review of the proceedings of the 1988 People First conference it was reported that people did not want to be labelled mentally handicapped; if people had to use a label they would prefer 'learning difficulties'. However, they wanted to be acknowledged as people first. In spite of the wishes of the People First movement the Department of Health has recently changed the terminology it uses from mental handicap to learning disability (McMillan 1991), thus effectively ignoring the consumers' views. Learning difficulty ensures that the emphasis is laid on the potential to learn rather than on a status quo label with an accent on the difference between people being of degree rather than of kind (Brechin and Swain 1988). Self reports from people labelled 'mentally handicapped' indicated that if they submitted to that term it validated their socially inferior status (Rhoades *et al.* 1986). Like a self-fulfilling prophecy (Ryan and Thomas 1980), people are perceived as incurably dependent and ineducable and in return they behave in ways which confirm these perceptions.

Self-advocacy as a term has comparatively recently taken root in psychiatric services, but in no other disadvantaged group. This may be because the challenge to the services is worthy of a special name; however, special activities imply that they only happen on special occasions, in special places by special people (Dowson 1990a)! The request for being viewed as people first is lost and a new label is being applied, as Wolfensberger indicated when a journal article had a photograph with the caption 'Three self-advocates having lunch', thus effectively negating the request to be seen as people first. Other people speaking out to assert their rights do not usually label themselves as doing a special activity, yet people with learning difficulties are called and refer to themselves as self-advocates (Dowson 1990a). The continuous use of this terminology suggests that the concept of self-advocacy still lies with the professionals and academics, who enjoy this language. Whilst people are cloaked in a label they will find their lives are prescribed and circumstanced by those with the power to attach the label (King's Fund 1985). People First is therefore important, as it forces others to recognise them as people first.

☐ **The role of the service worker**

In the western world there currently exist two models of services: the medical model and the educational model (Brechin and Swain 1988). People with learning difficulties were not asked their views (Dowson 1990a) as to which model of service they required, and the growing consumer movement, in the form of self-advocacy, has had little influence as yet on these strongly established professional traditions. Both models project the professional as the privileged holder of exclusive knowledge, confining people with learning difficulties to a dependent role. It would, however, be unfair to suggest that attitudes have not altered over the past twenty years and to ignore the influence that self-advocacy has played in achieving this (Dowson 1990a). An example of this is the normalisation principle, which was put into practice by these professionals interacting with the self-advocacy movement (see Chapter 1 for further information).

Shoultz (1985) states that we have responsibilities to provide new opportunities for people to learn skills which will empower them as they struggle for mastery over their own life and other broader issues. The responsibility lies with all service workers to provide these experiences for all people with learning difficulties. The relationship between service worker and.'client' should at least not be in conflict with the self-advocacy movement (Brechin and Swain 1988). The growth of this movement reflects the spirit of self-determination to throw off the 'dependency cloak' induced by the style of professional help. Self-advocacy should happen as and when people want it to, even if this frustrates the professional. Their role as service workers should not, however, be one of sitting back and waiting for it to happen (Dowson 1990a). The role should be that of enabling through choice and education and encouraging links with self-advocacy groups.

☐ **The role of the adviser**

There has been some evidence that some groups are not good at sustaining themselves and do not develop into self-advocates, and this usually depends on the initial support these people receive (Sines 1988). This is often provided by an adviser to the group. Ideally, the adviser should be someone outside the service, possibly linked to a citizen advocacy project. However, there will still exist a conflict in roles. Well-meaning advisers can become involved and inadvertently destroy or neutralise important issues. Well-intentioned organisations can cause problems for the users by using phrases such as 'doing self-advocacy today' or 'let us divide into groups for self-advocacy' (Dowson 1990b). Training is therefore essential to ensure advisers know when to intervene and when to hold back, encouraging independence and withdrawing swiftly (Dowson 1990a).

The voice of people with learning difficulties is not always strong and requires support to complement it. The adviser must be aware of the power they possess and acknowledge how easy it could be to apply pressure to get others to conform to their view. Power is the basic issue at stake, and whilst each side (that is the self-advocacy group and the service) manoeuvres either to gain or to hold on to power, the adviser is left in the middle ground. The power the adviser holds is recognised as being more than that held by people with learning difficulties. In an attempt to hide this, advisers may disempower themselves. This can have a terminal effect, as the passive role adopted saps the energy from the others in the group, and not using the power does not mean it is transferred elsewhere (Dowson 1990a). Rogers (1978) explains that people power only comes from the people themselves and when used properly it can help others without coercion or control and without sapping others' energy. At the other extreme, people power can corrupt, serving one's own ego. In the adviser's role this could lead to the use of people with learning difficulties for self-glorification. This can be seen in groups where people with learning difficulties hold the 'chair' but the adviser controls the agenda and discussion. One method of overcoming this maze of conflicts is for people with learning difficulties to provide advice to new or developing groups.

☐ **Achievements of self-advocacy**

True advocacy is more than just speaking out: it involves fervour and depth of feeling, vigour and vehemence (Williams and Shoultz 1982), and doing much more than is done routinely.

Self-advocacy has won political battles. In Lewisham, the self-advocacy group is involved on appointment boards and represents views on the borough day care planning team. The Avro Centre acquired student status for all people attending what traditionally would have been an adult training centre. People First are currently trying to address equal opportunity issues (Booth 1990). A group called Advocacy in Action, made up of members who have learning difficulties, disabilities and a disabled co-worker, join others in their area to provide an annual report called 'Working Together' and produce a magazine called *Enable*. They have also been successful in gaining representation on planning groups and are communicating directly with politicians. Access to this activity is usually very difficult for people with disabilities (Oliver 1990). Self-advocacy holds emotional and moral power and is a profoundly political movement in the broadest sense (Shoultz 1985), yet aims and achievements are often modest, with the organisation being operated by staff. The term self-advocacy has become part of the jargon of the services, and although one of the frequent complaints from people with learning difficulties is about the language used by service workers they are accepting the use of this term to describe what they are doing when they make these complaints. People with learning difficulties may continue to use this term to give their activities greater credibility in the eyes of the professionals (Dowson 1990a). Consequently, there exists a risk of not reaching beyond the services, and people involved lose their identity and are called self-advocates.

As discussed earlier, it is important that self-advocacy does not become a special activity, in order that people with learning difficulties are able to say what they think and are taken seriously all of the time. This will help to dispel the critics' view, that suggests that there is an elite group of people who do not speak for all people with learning difficulties but are only concerned with political manipulation (Shearer 1986). The able world forgets that democracy usually occurs with a small active political group representing the rest of the population. Other disparaging views suggest that people who self-advocate are not really handicapped and use this as an excuse to claim 'ours are not able to do that', denying the fact that expression can be at all levels, including non-verbal behaviour. It is obvious from this that service workers have not grasped the concept that self-advocacy is not just another subject on the curriculum, but that it permeates every aspect of the individual's life (Dowson 1990a).

☐ Training

Currently many services insist that people are trained to do self-advocacy or are sent to a self-advocacy group for therapeutic reasons. The creation of pre-self-advocacy training suggests that self-advocacy is identified as being something separate from ordinary living training. This appears to treat the skills required by self-advocacy as different from skills which are socially valuable to learn. Consequently it is perceived as preparation for an activity which is only undertaken by devalued people (Dowson 1990a). Pre-self-advocacy training implies people are unable to have rights and respect until they acquire what is judged to be the correct level of competence.

One approach to overcome these areas of concern is a course run by Skills for People, which commenced in 1983 (Rowe 1990). This group facilitates many courses and relies on unpaid volunteers with physical disabilities or learning difficulties. A minimum number of professionals are involved on the planning team. Due to the membership of this group, the courses are planned around issues which concern people with disabilities and not those defined by those who are not disabled. Instead of perpetuating the approach of knowledge being held by the professionals, this can be viewed as a growing alteration of vision to achieve equal rights.

☐ Effects of self-advocacy

Overall, the effects of self-advocacy are being felt in care reviews, selection panels and resource planning (Sines 1988). Shared Action Planning (Brechin and Swain 1987), consumer choice (DHSS 1989), partnership (Taylor 1986) (see Chapter 8 for further information on these issues), and gentle teaching (Brandon 1990a), are all indicators of change. Services which are not concerning themselves with supporting and facilitating the processes of self-advocacy should be questioned (Brechin and Swain 1988). The reluctance to form self-advocacy groups reflects how the services continually treat the users with little respect for their views and rights (Dowson 1990a). Resources should be made available for people to start their own groups if they wish to do so.

Although it is probably appropriate that professionals are not directly involved, they should be committed to act on the decisions made by self-advocacy groups (Sines 1988). Groups which do not have executive power are unable to influence decisions which are being made and are ineffective.

■ Citizen advocacy

□ Definition

Lay or citizen advocacy is comprised of the persuasive and supportive activities of a trained, selected and coordinated person either in a one-to-one situation or in a group (Sines 1988). The Camberwell citizen advocacy project views the activity as a partnership between two people (Hadley 1988), where the interests of the person with a learning difficulty are represented vigorously, as if they are their own, through this friendship and relationship. This relationship is developed over time with people who have not had the opportunity to integrate fully into their community and take up full citizenship.

□ Development of citizen advocacy

Traditionally, people with learning difficulties have lacked this type of support, partially due to their isolation and passivity (Sang & O'Brien 1984). A number of service providers find it difficult to grasp the concept that people with learning difficulties are equal citizens. In addition to this, a number of service workers continue to deny advocacy, seeing it as their own role, when the true cornerstone of this type of project should be its full independence from the services (Sang & O'Brien 1984).

The resistance to working with independent advocates is often masked by a concern that they may stir up trouble for the person they are meant to be helping. There is much suspicion within services and the advocate is perceived as a complainer, busybody, nuisance or spy (Blanch 1985). Social exclusion therefore continues, with people with learning difficulties only meeting their relatives or staff. Advocacy projects have to challenge the current systems and policies. Citizen advocacy can be the most exciting entity developing in our welfare state, and if it persists should be able to change policies which professionals and others have been unable to change (Sang & O'Brien 1984).

□ Citizen advocacy projects

To establish a project requires agreements and working relationships with all the services concerned. Sustaining these relationships is a noble aim; however, inevitable key problems in actual working practice arises (Sines 1988). To overcome distrust between professionals, parents and the advocate there needs to exist mutual understanding, confidence and trust. The Advocacy Alliance project operated from a centralised office; however, in order to improve its effectiveness it now seeks to move into local facilities. Law centres and Citizen's Advice Bureaux have been established in hospitals, but there is a danger that as they grow they may become an institution themselves. This would jeopardize the project, as it may start serving the needs of the organisation and not those of the clients or advocates. To safeguard against this happening a code of ethics for advocates is a valuable document. This code would act as a reminder of the essential planning which must accompany such projects (Sines 1988).

Sang & O'Brien (1984) stated that it is important that advocacy is defined early and clearly to enable the wider community to understand the functions of the project, as misinterpretation can be damaging to new proposals. Wolfensberger & Zauha (1973) described the role of an advocate as representing the instrumental and expressive needs of the person with learning difficulty. It is therefore important that the advocates are independent of the 'state' in order to avoid conflict of interests (Hadley 1988). In addition to this, loyalty to advocacy would remain paramount, serving the needs of the client in preference to the needs of the project or service. Advocates need to avoid gravitating towards being friends with the staff before the client.

Recruitment is a difficult exercise as it is difficult to identify potential advocates (Sines 1988), who are volunteers prepared to give significant commitment to this role. The advocate needs to be prepared to suffer the following costs: time, stress, money, sleep, leisure and pleasure. The advocate could also face resentment, hostility, ridicule and rejection (Sang & O'Brien 1984). This self-sacrificing vigour (Wolfensberger 1977) which is required means that there are low numbers of potential volunteers (Sang & O'Brien 1984).

Once advocates have been recruited it is important that they receive backing from an administrative machine, as this will provide the necessary stability. Without this, the voluntary efforts of an advocate will not have any major effects on the client's life. The office should be independent both financially and organisationally from the service provider (Wolfensberger 1977; Hadley 1988), and the citizen advocate must not supplement the workforce. Advocates are not volunteers to the service (Carle 1984); they exist to protect the rights of the client.

Advertising for advocates needs to be carried out with much thought. It is essential that it is carried out in such a way that it projects a valued image of people with learning difficulties. Volunteers need to be screened, as they frequently adopt a sympathetic view to the client group which is demeaning in two ways. Firstly, it implies that it requires special people to take on this role, and secondly, it suggests a one-sided relationship, with the client being the passive recipient of benevolence (Sang & O'Brien 1984). One method of overcoming this is to establish community networks which will respond to providing friendship, and a local office can facilitate this.

☐ **Friendship**

Befriending occurs when a valued person links up with another to share skills, interests and experiences. Befriending schemes and citizen advocacy have given people with learning difficulties the opportunity to make friends with a person who is not a member of staff or a relative. Frequently, people with learning difficulties are required to rely solely on disabled peers for support, which often exaggerates their difficulties. The act of developing and retaining friendships can be quite a complicated challenge (see Chapter 5 for more information). The choice of friend can influence whether an individual's self-identity will be stigmatised. This depends on whether they select a disabled peer or a socially valued relationship with a non-handicapped person (Rhoades *et al.* 1986). Kaufmann (1984) indicated that the social opportunities for people with learning difficulties are limited. These opportunities are frequently provided in special facilities, and only a few people made reciprocal friends who were non-handicapped. In contrast to this, research found that these people wanted close, intimate friendships (Booth 1990), and saw such friendships as lacking from their life. Citizen advocacy projects have been helpful in providing increased opportunities for people to extend their social contacts.

It is commonly believed that staff or parents could be developing their role to include that of a friend. However, there is a conflict of interest retained by these parties. No one individual is an expert in being an ordinary citizen (King's Fund 1988), and non-service workers are ideally placed to raise issues in relation to people with learning difficulties, without causing too much conflict in the friendship.

In contrast to the view that families cannot be advocates, the Rowntree Trust established a disability programme to empower families. This approach was taken as it was felt that there existed a lack of consultation when discussing the change from hospital to community care. The United Kingdom does not readily involve service users or their families in the development of services. This is in contrast to Canada and America, where they are viewed as an important coalition for change. Parents and service users in the United Kingdom are now speaking with greater force to be included in the discussions about service development (Booth 1990).

☐ **Effects of citizen advocacy**

Advocacy is not an easy skill to assimilate into practice. It requires training for all participants (Sines 1988). Advocacy projects are increasing throughout the United Kingdom and they are having an impact on services. Quality assurance projects which use service accomplishments (see Chapters 2 and 8) ensure clients receive an acceptable standard of service. Supportive partnerships (Carle 1984) provide a change in the belief that people with learning difficulties need things done for them to one that shares activities and interests with them.

Service brokerage, a Canadian led approach, empowers individuals, with technical support and advice, to make effective use of their allocation of funds. The primary objective is to enable people with learning difficulties to participate fully in the community with control and empowerment (Brandon 1990b). Case management, designed to provide individual packages of care to meet the person's needs is implicit in the 'Caring for People' document (Department of Health 1989; see Chapter 1).

Case management can promote consumerism by various methods (PSSRU 1990). Safeguards will be necessary to ensure that clients' needs and wishes remain central to ensure that consumer choice becomes a reality (Audit Commission 1989). However, as case management has not become mandatory it could be suggested that it is not a high priority on the political agenda (Barker & Peck 1990). Access to independent advocates can act as a safeguard to ensure that clients' wishes and views are maintained on the political agenda.

■ Conclusion

There exists a host of historical, social and political reasons why people who live 'in care' are often treated as if they were less valuable than other human beings (Sang & O'Brien 1984). The spectrum of advocacy movements and the everyday activities of people with learning difficulties can change this. However, this requires services which are prepared to create supportive environments which enhance the empowerment process, and to listen to the consumer's voice. The use of jargon in documents, reports and legislation ensures that the professionals remain in control, as service users do not understand this language. People First states that it would like professionals to stop using labels. However, it continues to use the term 'self-advocacy' which suggests that the power held by the service workers has not been relinquished (see Chapter 8).

The concept of advocacy and the parallel concept of social role valorisation (Wolfensberger 1988) requires radically different thinking with regard to the revision of the role of the professional and service worker approach. When people who have previously not had a voice begin to speak, there is good reason to be excited and inspired. There is growing pressure on professionals and service workers to surrender their power and control and recognise the inherent problems of the attitudes and practices which promote rather than reduce dependency in clients. Professional debate should be informed by advocacy groups' opinions in the future. Experiences and thoughts of the users will become directly available to decision makers; however, they are required to listen.

■ Reference

Audit Commission (1989). *Developing community care for adults with a mental handicap*. Occasional Paper, 9 October. HMSO, London.

Barker, I. & Peck, E. (1990). Snakes and ladders. *Insight*, 9 May, 20–1.

Blanch, R. (1985). Citizen advocacy. *Nursing Mirror*. 3 April.

Booth, T. (1990). Better lives: Changing services for people with learning difficulties. *Social Services Monographs: Research in practice*. CCETSW, London.

Brandon, D. (1990a). Gentle teaching. *Nursing Times*. **86** (2), 62–3.

Brandon, D. (1990b). Editorial comments. *Community Living*. April.

Brechin, A. & Swain, J. (1987). *Changing relationships. Shared action planning with people with mental handicap*. Harper & Row, London.

Brechin, A. & Swain, J. (1988). Professional/client relationships: Creating a working alliance with people with learning difficulties. *Disability, Handicap and Society*. 3 March.

Carle, N. (1984). *Key concepts in the community based services*. CMH Publications, London.

Department of Health (1989). *Caring for people. Community care in the next decade and beyond*. HMSO, London.

DHSS (1971). *Better services for the mentally handicapped*. HMSO, London.

Dowson, S. (1990a). *Keeping it safe. Self-advocacy by people with learning difficulties and the professional response. Challenge to consensus*. Values into Action, London.

Dowson, S. (1990b). Why not let self-advocacy spreak for itself? *Community Living*. 9 October.

Hadley, J. (1988). Speaking for one and all. *Community Care*. 27 September, 145–6.

Kaufman, S. (1984). Friendship coping systems and community adjustment of mildly retarded adults. Cited in *Rhoades et al. (1986) Rehabilitation Literature*. **47** (1–2), 2–7.

King's Fund (1985). *Advocacy and people with long term disabilities. A report of a conference held at the King's Fund Centre*. King Edward's Hospital Fund for London.

King's Fund (1988). *Ties and connections: An ordinary community life for people with learning difficulties*. King Edward's Hospital Fund for London.

McMillan, I. (1991). Dorrell pledges RNMHs will not be discarded. *Nursing Times*. 3 July. **87** (27), 7.

Oliver, M. (1990). *The politics of disablement*. Macmillan Education Ltd, Basingstoke.

PSSRU (1990). Lessons from a demonstration programme. *Care in the Community*. 9 May PSSRU, University of Kent.

Rhoades, C., Browning, P. & Thorn, E. (1986). Self help advocacy movement: A promised peer support system for people with mental disability. *Rehabilitation Literature*. **47** (1–2), 2–7.

Rogers, C. (1978). *Carl Rogers on personal power*. Constable, London.

Rowe, N. (1990). A sense of pride. *Community Living*. April.

Ryan, J. & Thomas, P. (1980). *The politics of mental handicap*. Penguin, Harmondsworth.
Sang, B. & O'Brien, J. (1984). *Advocacy: the UK and American experience*. King's Fund project paper 51. King Edward's Hospital Fund for London.
Shearer, A. (1986). *Building communities*. Oxford University Press, Oxford.
Shoultz, B. (1985). Making it work through self-advocacy *CMH Newsletter*. **40** (Spring), 9.
Sines, D. (ed.) (1988). *Towards integration: Comprehensive services for people with mental handicaps*. Harper & Row, London.
Taylor, J. (1986). *Mental handicap: Partnership in the community*. Office of Health Economics/Mencap, London.
United Nations (1971). *Declaration of rights of mentally retarded persons*. General Assembly Resolution 2856 (XXVI).
Williams, P. & Shoultz, B. (1982). *We can speak for ourselves*. Souvenir, London.
Wolfensberger, W. (1972). *The principle of normalisation in human services*. National Institute of Mental Retardation, Toronto.
Wolfensberger, W. (1977). *A multi-component advocacy and protection schema*. Canadian Association of Mental Retardation, Toronto.
Wolfensberger, W. (1988). Social role valorisation: A proposed new term for the principle of normalisation. *Mental Retardation*. **35** (6), 234–9.
Wolfensberger, W. & Zauha, H. (1973). *Citizen advocacy*. National Institute of Mental Retardation, Toronto.

Chapter 5

Personal relationships

Patricia Brigden

■ Introduction

As stated in Chapter 1, the underpinning philosophy of many services is that of normalisation.

As more adults with learning difficulties are expected to lead 'normalised' lifestyles so the need to develop a shared view in society about their personal relationships becomes an increasingly urgent priority. Historically, this subject has largely been ignored. Men and women were segregated, resulting in an increased incidence of homosexual behaviour in old Victorian-style institutions. With modern care practices this segregation is no longer a possibility. Adults with learning difficulties have rights and increasingly know that they have these rights. They wish to and are encouraged to exercise choice in the type of relationships they develop.

The expression of these rights may cause difficulties to service providers. The following case example illustrates a common dilemma. John was referred to the Community Mental Handicap Team for inappropriately touching women in an indiscriminate way on the bus transporting trainees to and from the day service placement. Community Mental Handicap Team staff included John in sex education classes during which he learned that it might be more appropriate to acquire himself a girlfriend and restrict intimate touching to that relationship. John was successful in developing such a relationship and this was satisfactory for about one year. One day John approached the Community Mental Handicap Team and said it was time to develop the relationship but he needed help in finding a suitable private place. This proved to be a problem that staff were not able to help with at the time. Prior to staff offering the requested help the legal aspects had to be considered. The issue of how much support staff could expect from the senior managers, who did not have the appropriate knowledge and expertise, also needed to be addressed. Resolving these issues was likely to be a long-term task. Failure to help, however, in this case may have been one of the causative factors which led this young man to commit a sexual offence and end up on a section of the Mental Health Act (DHSS 1983b).

This chapter considers the fact that people with learning difficulties have the same sexual feelings and needs as other citizens. They can and do make satisfactory relationships. This chapter also addresses the issues regarding the general public's attitudes to the expression of sexuality by people with learning difficulties and promotes the notion that sexual relations are acceptable. Effective sex education should be consistently provided in special schools and day service placements, as this will help people with learning difficulties to cope with their own sexuality and to be more responsible as they gain greater freedom of action. There is a growing body of experiential evidence that people with learning difficulties can enter into and sustain stable and satisfactory marriages (Craft & Craft 1979). Guidance on contraception is supplied by the Family Planning Association (Dixon 1986) and bodies such as the Brooke Advisory Centre have pioneered information leaflets which require a minimum of literacy to be understood. There is still considerable debate about whether a couple with learning difficulties should produce children, the main concern being for the child. Will the child receive adequate care? There is an urgent requirement for developing policy informed by lively debate and taking into account legal considerations in local areas. In view of the climate of change, this should be kept under constant review. Organisations such as MIND have produced useful guidelines on subject areas to be included in policy (MIND 1982).

When considering personal relationships, it should be remembered that a great deal other than sexual activity deserves consideration. Adults with learning difficulties, their parents and carers need to focus their attention on the wider subject of warm, caring personal relationships and how they might be achieved. (Quest for Improvement Ltd 1992).

Gradually, throughout childhood, people learn to know how other people are feeling and to respond appropriately. They learn about different types of relationship. They develop positive self-esteem and ways to protect themselves. There is common agreement on when, how and where it is appropriate to touch other people. These rules of society are gradually taught and assimilated by the growing child, who gains knowledge from school, friends, TV, parents, reading and films. Parents protect less as the child develops, and start to encourage independence, though continuing to support and guide as necessary. Some risk-taking is inevitable. At 18 years the child legally becomes an adult, with rights and responsibilities. Parents hope that at this stage enough has been learned for the new young adult to be socially acceptable, to be able to take sensible decisions that harm neither the person nor others and that he or she will have satisfying personal relationships enabling a full life to be led (Quest for Improvement Ltd 1991).

■ Social interaction

People spend considerable amounts of time engaged in social interaction. This is because social interaction underpins how society and the community function. It provides us with our pleasure and satisfaction. It is a powerful and effective social reinforcer.

Common social reinforcers used include making eye contact, paying attention and smiling when appropriate. Positive and negative messages must be expressed effectively and in such a way that both the person sending the message and the person receiving it feel safe. Any situation calls for a specific social skill. A person needs to use the right skill in the right situation, thus requiring coordination. To illustrate this requirement, one only has to think of situations where the verbal signal must be supported by the non-verbal signals. If this does not happen the person is read as insincere. Use of social skills tends to be automatic and unconscious. Despite this they are learned behaviours which require practise. Social skills affect our interactions. They also affect how we are perceived and valued by others.

Adults with learning difficulties need assistance to become more valued members of society. It is important to help them improve their social effectiveness in order to achieve this. It is recognised that people with learning difficulties can and do learn new skills, albeit slowly. Their social skills constitute an important topic to be incorporated both into formal curricula (schools, further education, day services) and into individual programme plans (IPPs).

In response to need a number of training programmes have been developed (Graves Medical Audiovisual Library). They tend to deal with subjects such as social skills training for people with lesser or greater degrees of learning difficulties. There is a need to demonstrate the importance of social skills to ordinary living, to identify the commonly encountered types of skills deficits, to indicate how practical training sessions may be run to teach skills, and to emphasise how essential regular practice of skills is. It follows from this that opportunities must be generated if skills are to be maintained and generalised.

When considering the importance of social skills to adults with learning difficulties it is essential to ensure the skills meet the needs of the clients. People with learning difficulties generally have poor social interaction skills. Ordinary people therefore do not interact with them because of paucity of response. There is therefore a need to increase their social skills, but it is difficult to break into the vicious circle. The following may be a suitable course of action: start with simple work on basic skills, such as eye contact, paying attention, turn-taking and so on. Some of the known obstacles in the way of learning social skills are physical handicaps and/or speech disorders, which make interaction difficult. Both physiotherapists and speech therapists may have helpful advice to offer here (see Chapter 9). Occasionally it is the poor social environment which fails to provide either opportunities to learn new skills and/or to practise existing skills. In institutional settings staff frequently tell residents what to do rather than interacting with them. The result is a group of residents showing few signs of awareness of others, let alone showing even basic ideas about interaction. Likewise, in community settings many people do not know how to behave in relation to people with learning difficulties and so avoid them. Situations likely to promote learning are therefore reduced.

To facilitate learning among adults with severe learning difficulties some principles should be followed. Programmes need to be highly structured. Sessions must be short to allow for poor concentration. It is important never to underestimate a person's capacity to learn. Lots of time to learn and lots of opportunities to practise skills should be constantly and regularly provided. Teaching sessions should be stimulating and enjoyable. It is most effective if the outcome is meaningful to the client, for example if he or she cooks something and then eats it. Staff and carers need to be involved to ensure their awareness and to encourage them to enable everyday practice of skills for the clients. Everybody involved will need constant reminders of the importance of practice and rewards for achieving targeted skills and for making reasonable attempts.

Early research showed that activity groups could be successfully used to develop skills, but it was also shown they made little impact on real life. To ensure that new behaviour is so thoroughly learned that it is maintained, and also is seen to occur in new situations, skills must be practised in real-life situations. It is possible to utilise naturally occurring situations such as work, leisure, domestic and social activities.

When Williams *et al.* (1989) looked at using mealtimes to develop social interaction, they concluded that it was essential that people with learning difficulties live in a social environment that promotes the development and use of social skills. The importance of leisure activities as a context in which personal relationships may be initiated and fostered is elaborated on in Chapter 6. Finally, carers and staff need to examine their own behaviour with the severely handicapped to ensure that they are recognising and acting on some of the subtle ways people may be attempting to use to interact, e.g. eye contact, sounds, expressions and emotions.

To interact successfully in society a person needs to be assertive, have positive self-esteem and to be able to protect him- or herself. To commence discussing these kinds of issue with clients, carers can explore the degree of understanding of the different types of relationship which exist. Clients could be assisted in breaking down their family relationships into parent–child, brother–sister, uncle–niece, cousins, first cousin once removed and so on. The scale of intimacy from stranger to acquaintance, colleague (working relationship), friend, good friend or lover can be explored. Heterosexual and homosexual variations on the theme can be explored, and marriage and parenthood require elaboration.

It is essential that adults with mild learning difficulties are fully conversant with the concept of friendship and what this means. They need to be able to demonstrate that they understand that friendship is a two-way process, involving give and take, and that certain types of behaviour are appropriate to certain levels of intimacy, such as kissing.

When examining the appropriateness of behaviour in a relationship a number of aspects need to be considered. These are:

- The social acceptability of touch in different situations.

- Knowing the difference between public and private places.

- Respecting personal space.

- Responding to introductions appropriately.

Dealing with feelings and emotions appropriately requires a range of subtle and sophisticated skills. These are:

- Naming range of emotions correctly, e.g. fear, anger and so on.

- Ability to read facial expressions, body language and tone of voice.

- Controlling own feelings (When do you show your feelings? How strongly do you show them?).

- Verbal expression of feelings.

- Use of matching body language.

It will be apparent by this stage that in addition to teaching 'behaviours', aspects such as perception and cognition are critically important to effective social interaction. Looking and listening, getting information from others and reading the social situation are all essential. Planning, problem solving and evaluating are also important to effective functioning; for example what does a person decide to do when they have to consider how to attract someone's attention in a crowded room in a socially acceptable way (Brigden & Keleher 1990)? Successful teaching methods used with adults with learning difficulties include verbal and written instructions, modelling, role play and homework. There is a growing amount of material around to help staff and carers to teach about aspects of personal relationships (Craft 1982; Craft & Craft 1982). The Kempton slides (Kempton & Hanson 1978) are an example of an attempt to provide a comprehensive package of slide material from which selection can be made to cover topics and/or to suit individuals or groups. These slides cover the following areas: parts of the body; male puberty; female puberty; social behaviours; human reproduction; birth control; venereal disease and sexual health; marriage; and parenting. There are examples of comprehensive packages of slide material which can be drawn from to assist with individual assessment and educational sessions. In addition, some work has been conducted on what could be usefully included in teaching social skills to people with severe learning difficulties (Brigden *et al.* 1990).

■ Attitudes

To achieve a rich social environment, staff, carers, parents and the general public need to understand the special needs of people with learning difficulties and to change their behaviour and attitudes so that they facilitate appropriate social interaction.

The right to appropriate sexual expression is a continuation of the philosophy of normalisation (Wolfensberger 1972). Though recent surveys suggest the attitudes of staff are moving in a more liberal direction (Johnson & Davies 1989) it is felt that attitudes may not be put into practice because of feelings of inadequacy or ambivalence. If this is a problem in relation to heterosexual behaviour, it is a greater one where homosexual behaviour is concerned; even in these enlightened times, both staff and parents may be prejudiced or fear others' reaction to homosexuality. Staff's personal attitudes towards contraception and abortion can also prevent effective decision-making. If staff have difficulties discussing heterosexual relationships with parents it can be more difficult break to the news that their son or daughter is involved in a homosexual relationship, for the reasons already stated. These problems help explain why some staff err on the side of excessive caution and find themselves controlling people's relationships. Unfortunately, such staff still have a disproportionate influence on practice.

Programmes and activities to train staff have been published (Stevens *et al.* 1988), but there has been no clear advice given on the amount and type of training needed to effect a significant change of attitudes. It is therefore interesting to note findings by Rose & Holmes (1991), who evaluated one-day and three-day staff training workshops and found some positive attitude change after one day's training and significant ($p<0.001$) attitude change after three days' training. An attitude inventory adapted from Brantlinger (1983, 1987) was used to assess degree of change. The authors conclude that more work is needed to identify which components of the training proved effective.

■ The law

It has become increasingly recognised that staff need a policy or guidelines to help them respond to the sexuality of clients with learning difficulties. Many statutory agencies, voluntary agencies and organisations in the private sector are in the process of devising policy. The main concern is to do with legal liability. The law as it relates to people with learning difficulties is at best confusing and at times unsatisfactory. Few people are really clear on the issues. There are a number of lawyers around who have become interested in guiding the layperson through the complexities of the law. Though there are few clear-cut answers to individual questions, there are some critical questions that need to be considered (Carson 1987). These questions probe for possible transgressions of laws which were devised to tackle the following issues:

- Negligence.

- Underage sexual activity.

- Exploitation.

- Ability to consent.

- Protection of a client's civic or legal rights.

- Trespass.

- Incitement.

- Vicarious or direct liability of employers for civil offences of their employees.

The law of negligence applies where there is a duty of care, that is if a client is in receipt of a service which meets personal needs. If the answer 'yes' follows the question 'Can you *reasonably* foresee that your action or inaction, or the action of your client might cause harm to the client or others?' then there is a duty of care. It is possible therefore to know about a problem, ignore it, and be guilty of negligence. It is easy therefore to see that staff are operating in a grey area where sometimes it is neither all right to take action nor all right not to take it. It is to be hoped that formally organised policy and guidelines will clarify the positions that staff all too frequently find themselves in.

The law goes by biological age. An individual must be over 16 years to consent to heterosexual acts and 21 years to consent to male homosexual acts (Dixon & Gunn 1985).

There is great anxiety to ensure that people with learning difficulties are not exploited. The safest line of action is to appear to be meeting the client's goals and to be accepting his or her values. If the answer to the question 'Who benefits from an intervention?' is other than the client, i.e. staff, service or family, there could be a concern that the client is being exploited.

When considering whether a client is legally able to consent to sexual activity, the case hinges on whether a person with an arrested or incomplete development of mind has severely impaired intelligence and/or severely impaired social functioning. (Intelligence quotients are not legally prescribed.) If the person does not, is adequately informed and is not subject to duress, then the person can consent. If there is severe impairment, then the court will wish to know if efforts are being made to improve the level of social functioning. Failure to do so could cause concern about whether the client's needs were being adequately met. The importance of trying to enhance an individual's level of social functioning is that while the client is severely impaired in social functioning his or her legal and civil rights are restricted.

Having established that a client is able to consent, he or she must know what is being consented to. It is therefore important that clients have had everything explained to them in a manner which they can comprehend. Alternative forms of communication can be used where appropriate, e.g. written explanations or sign language to a deaf and dumb person. It needs to be proved that the benefits and harms of any given course of action have been spelled out as appropriate. Each individual should be told as much as he or she wants to know. The client may automatically assent to everything. Attention needs to be paid to ensuring that people with learning difficulties are able to say 'no' when propositioned. This is best tackled with assertiveness training, which can be built into more generalised social skills training. The client also needs to have experienced a service which respects decisions made by clients. If this is not the case the client's rights may be seen to be infringed.

The law is concerned about the nature of the partner in sexual activity. It is a criminal offence when certain employees have sexual intercourse with certain female clients. It is illegal if sexual touching occurs with an individual unable to give his or her consent (i.e. those with severely impaired social functioning). Such a case can be defended if it is argued that the accused did not know the partner was severely impaired. In potential situations like this it may be helpful to advise a client that their intended partner may be incapable of giving legal consent. Touching a client may result in the law of trespass being involved. Defences to trespass are (1) consent and (2) the argument that it was social touching (Carson 1987; Dixon & Gunn 1985).

The service has a duty to spell out for clients what behaviours are expected to take place in private. Staff should be adequately trained and supported by their employers. Employers have a duty to advise employees how to respond to clients' sexuality and to provide them with appropriate support in doing so. If it can be proved that this was not the case, and that a client or employee came to harm, the employer would be directly liable. Staff are expected to respond to client needs even if this is against their own personal values (e.g. views on contraception and abortion).

The above review of how the law is likely to react to cases made in the area of personal relationships indicates an uncertain situation. There is scope for the court and jury to make interpretations in grey areas. It is therefore helpful for staff to be kept aware of the law. This is a changing field. The law commissioners are currently reviewing aspects of the law relating to this subject (DHSS 1991). Regardless of any changes, it is essential to have a formal local policy. The importance of 'formal' is that senior managers are aware of the issues, and have made certain decisions about what behaviours they expect from their staff in what situations, and thus when and to what degree they are likely to give their support.

■ The need for policy and guidelines for carers

A great deal has already been said about the need for a formal local policy and guidelines for staff. The following practical guidance may provide a useful framework for policy development.

1. Working toward shared values throughout the organisation from care assistants to managers.

2. Identification of the current position in a service/organisation via assessment. The assessor must have positive attitudes.

3. Is the assessor the only person in the organisation with the right attitudes? Do other staff have similar attitudes who can be supportive?

4. If there are supportive staff then are these among managers or direct care staff or a mixture of both? Are the majority in support, or only a minority?

The answers to these questions will suggest what should be done next. Sometimes workshops or staff training sessions can start to address the issue, while sometimes inputs through committees or powerful opinion leaders can trigger a chain of events that set the organisation moving in the right direction. A recent initiative in this direction was to arrange a meeting of all interested parties, the outcome of which was not only quarterly meetings to build a support network (a horizontal strategy), but an action plan which included collaboration to lay on a workshop for top managers (a vertical strategy). Though this stage is slow, and frustrating for advanced thinkers, it is essential to get everyone to the point where they understand the issues and own the proposed solutions. Unless this is the case, any policy produced will merely gather dust on a shelf.

The purpose of policy is to empower and enable staff to support people with learning difficulties in their personal relationships. Policy also acts as a safeguard to prevent exploitation both of staff and clients. A good policy accepts that an element of risk is inevitable in this area. Risks are best faced up to by shared decision-making in multidisciplinary case discussions. If management formally accepts the multidisciplinary case discussion as the forum for clinical decisions about aspects of personal relationships, then staff have an effective support mechanism.

Modern policy should not be paternalistic. Early attempts at policy led to rules such as the following one 'The couple should be going out for X times before they can hold hands'. Since ordinary members of the community do not have to abide by such rules, neither should people with learning difficulties.

It is generally felt that guidelines need to give consideration to the

following areas: bodily development; masturbation; petting; sexual intercourse; contraception; sterilisation and vasectomies; cohabitation and marriage; parenthood; unwanted pregnancy; homosexuality; pornography; and
sexually transmitted diseases (Mind 1982). Guidelines need to cover aspects
such as the personal rights of clients (including in some cases for protection
from unwanted advances), risk-taking and opportunities, how to get decisions made and the principle of least restrictive practice. The potential
role of an advocate in these circumstances could be outlined. (This has been
covered in detail in Chapter 4.) The question of how much parents can or
should influence decisions needs to be covered. A view on the personal
moral standards of staff should be set out, including the position on staff
relationships with clients. The requirements of the law should be covered.
Reference needs to be made to relevant sections of the Sexual Offences Act
and the Mental Health Act. The guidelines need to facilitate staff in their
attempts to gain advice on the law. Related areas should be incorporated,
such as sex education, individual programme planning systems and ethical
and ethnic issues. The needs and attitudes of staff needs to be acknowledged
and catered for. Last, but not least, the guidelines should be given a context
which is embedded in service philosophy and principles (East Berkshire
Health Authority 1990; Basingstoke and North Hampshire Health Authority 1990). Clients, staff, parents and agencies all need a policy to guide
their professional practice. A shared policy will greatly aid liaison between
agencies and groupings.

■ Counselling parents

It has already been mentioned that guidelines for staff need to consider how
much parents can or should influence decisions made about their son or
daughter's personal relationships.

As children grow up, parents naturally go through a process of letting
go and allowing or enabling their sons and daughters to make their own
decisions and take responsibility for their own actions. Most parents have
some problems trying not to be overprotective, and in deciding the
appropriate level of risk-taking that should be permitted. These problems
are exaggerated where the son or daughter has learning difficulties. It is
generally a difficult task to successfully learn to gradually let go and empower a son or daughter to take his or her own decisions. Many parents fail
in achieving this step and long-term overprotection can result. It is not
uncommon to find retired people with sons or daughters at home in their
forties and fifties who are never allowed to be in the house alone for half an
hour, let alone have relationships, and where it is clear that the person, if
perceived as a capable adult, could be considerably more independent than
they are ever allowed to be. This can be a cause of challenging behaviour as

the adult with learning difficulties struggles against a world in which he or she is perceived as a 'child' and told what he or she can and cannot do.

In view of the difficulties faced by parents in terms of letting go, they may be concerned about their son or daughter developing relationships. Staff may require assistance to work with parents, who typically display signs of anxiety about relationships. It is important when discussing relationships with parents to find out exactly what is worrying them. An example was Mrs Heyes who explained she thought her daughter Mary should not go out with John (a friend from the day service placement) in the evenings. When asked why not, she said Mary could not cope with marriage and babies and she was desperately afraid of unwanted pregnancy. In this case it was possible to explore these concerns in relation to Mary and John's individual situation. Did Mrs Heyes feel so bad about the relationship if pregnancy was not an issue? Mrs Heyes replied that she felt much better about it. Did Mrs Heyes feel Mary would cope with a contraception method? Yes, she did, and help could be supplied with this. Did Mrs Heyes feel the relationship between John and Mary had reached this stage? Her response was 'no'. Mrs Heyes was told that they would both understand and benefit from sex education which could be supplied, and she began to relax and see that if life was approached in a systematic, step-by-step but proactive manner, Mary could have a fulfilled and satisfying relationship which would benefit all concerned, including Mrs Heyes herself, who would have time to herself when John and Mary were out. By systematic problem analysis it is frequently possible to demonstrate to parents that many of their anxieties and worries are not as great as they feared. This is experienced as very reassuring by parents.

Common concerns expressed by parents are:

- They are unable to cope for themselves so they can't marry.

- They could not care for a baby so they must not have one.

- They won't cope with contraception methods.

Though most people respond positively to a counselling approach, there is the occasional parent who cannot be shifted from a totally negative point of view. In this case it may be necessary to supply the individual with an advocate. (Advocacy is explored in Chapter 4.)

■ Social support networks

In response to 'Care in the community' (DHSS 1983a), and 'An ordinary life' (King's Fund 1980), and as a way of putting into practice the principles of normalisation (e.g. Tyne 1981), many group homes for people with learning difficulties have opened.

It was generally thought that by living in 'ordinary houses' greater opportunities would be created for community participation, integration and formation and maintenance of social relationships. All of these features are thought to indicate an improved quality of life for the individual.

In recent years there has been interest in evaluating these assumptions (McConkey *et al.* 1983).

• Is quality of life better in a small ordinary house?

• Is better social integration achieved?

• What contact is there with 'ordinary people'?

• What use is made of community facilities such as pubs, clubs and shops?

Social support plays a key role in enabling people with learning difficulties to live as independently as possible (Edgerton *et al.* 1984). Too often the support is provided by a formal network of professionals and volunteers. This support tends to be unequal in that a carer is assisting a 'client'. It seems probable that relationships initiated by people with learning difficulties are more beneficial (Donegan & Potts 1988).

Relationships are perceived by people with learning difficulties as strongly related to 'quality of life' (Edgerton 1967). Research indicates that a lower percentage of people with learning difficulties living in group homes have 'special friends', despite this being a recognised quality of life indicator.

Heggs (1988) followed up on an ex-hospital resident who moved out into a group home to see how the social network developed over the first few months after the move. She looked at the number, type and duration of activities and contacts with family and other non-handicapped people. Social support functions looked at were (Barrera & Ainley 1983):

• Material aid, e.g. going to bank.

• Behavioural assistance, e.g. sharing tasks.

• Intimate interaction, e.g. someone listening to individual.

• Guidance, e.g. being offered advice.

• Feedback.

• Positive social interaction (for fun and relaxation).

The client went out more than he had in hospital, but the range of community facilities used was quite limited. Factors such as the client's limited mobility and the newness of staff who were not local and did not know the area were seen to limit the extent of community usage. Contact with local residents was limited to talking over the fence and similar interactions of short duration. Family contact increased (as others, such as De Kock *et al.* (1985), have found). Generally speaking it seems the social network of an individual with learning difficulties tends to be dependent on the main care-provider. Thus staff working in group homes need to be selected for their interest in encouraging interaction with local networks (Firth 1987). If this is not done, the group home and the individuals in it could be potentially more isolated than in a hospital setting, thereby defeating the aims of community care and 'normalisation'.

When staffing group homes, training programmes need to include orientation to the facilities in a locality and information relating to volunteer agencies.

When volunteers regularly accompany people with learning difficulties to evening classes or to leisure and sports outings, friendships are more likely to develop. It is necessary to meet many people as acquaintances in many different settings to provide a context in which friendships may materialise (Firth 1987).

Friendship involves reciprocal liking. In small group houses staff and residents form close relationships. There needs to be more research done on the emotional effects that could occur when staff leave, especially in situations where staff played a significant role in the social network.

■ Summary

The majority of personal relationships are not of a sexual nature. It is up to staff and carers to find out what kinds of relationship clients want with their peers and to enable and facilitate these to happen. There is a lot of unnecessary anxiety about close friendships where the last thing on the clients' minds is physical intimacy. Too often relationships are broken up in the fear it may develop into intimate behaviour. This of course often leads to entirely understandable behaviour problems and/or grieving.

■ References

Barrera, M. & Ainley, S. L. (1983). The structure of social support: A conceptual and empirical analysis. *Journal of Community Psychology*. II, 133–43.
Basingstoke and North Hampshire Health Authority (1990). *Sexuality of people with a mental handicap. Guidelines for staff.*
Brantlinger, E. (1983). Measuring variation and change in attitudes of residential

care staff toward the sexuality of mentally retarded persons. *Mental retardation.* **21**, 17–22.

Brantlinger, E. (1987). Influencing staff attitudes. In *Mental handicap and sexuality issues and perspectives* (ed. A. Craft). Costello, Tunbridge Wells.

Brigden, P. & Keleher, R. (1990). *Social skills training and people with mild mental handicap.* Graves Medical Audiovisual Library (Cat No. 87/17/G), Cheltenham.

Brigden, P., Keleher, R. & Tyson, J. (1990). *Social skills training for people with severe mental handicap.* Graves Medical Audiovisual Library (Cat. No. 87/26/G), Cheltenham.

Carson, D. (1987). *The law and the sexuality of people with a mental handicap.* University of Southampton, Southampton.

Craft, A. (1982). *Health and hygiene and sex education for mentally handicapped children, adolescents and adults.* Health Education Council's Resource Centre, 71–75 New Oxford Street, London WC1A 1AH.

Craft, M. & Craft, A. (1982). *Sex and the mentally handicapped. A guide for parents and carers.* Routledge & Kegan Paul, London.

Craft, A. & Craft, A. (1979). *Handicapped married couples. A Welsh study of couples handicapped from birth by mental, physical, or personality disorder.* Routledge, London.

De Kock, U., Felce, D., Saxby, H. & Thomas, H. (1985). *Community and family contact: An evaluation of small community homes for severely and profoundly mentally handicapped adults.* Health Care Evaluation Research Team, University of Southampton, Southampton.

DIISS (1983a) *Care in the community.* HMSO, London.

DHSS (1983b) *Mental Health Act.* HMSO, London.

DHSS (1991). *The Law Commission consultation paper 119 Mentally incapacitated adults and decision making: An overview.* HMSO, London.

Dixon, H. (1986). *Options for change.* Family Planning Association, London.

Dixon, H. & Gunn, M. (1985). *Sex and the law. A brief guide for staff working in the mental handicap field.* Family Planning Association, London.

Donegan, C. & Potts, M. (1988). People with mental handicap living alone in the community. A pilot study of their quality of life. *British Journal of Mental Subnormality* **35** 1(66), 10–22.

East Berkshire Health Authority (1990). *Personal Relationships.*

Edgerton, R. B., Bollinger, M. & Herr, B. (1984). The cloak of competence: after two decades. *American Journal of Mental Deficiency.* **88**, 345–51.

Edgerton, R. B., Bollinger, M. & Herr, B. (1984). The cloak of competence: after two decades. *American Journal of Mental Deficiency.* **88**, 345–51.

Firth, H. (1987). A move from hospital to community: evaluation of community contacts. *Child Care, Health and Development.* **13** (5), 341–53.

Heggs, A. (1988). *Social support networks among people with learning difficulties.* (unpublished).

Johnson, P. R. & Davies, R. (1989). Sexual attitudes of members of staff. *British Journal of Mental Subnormality.* **35**, 17–21.

Kempton, W. & Hanson, G. (1978). *Sexuality and the mentally handicapped. Nine slide presentations for teaching the mentally handicapped individual* (2nd edn). Distributed by SFA Santa Monica, California.

King's Fund (1980). *An ordinary life: Comprehensive locally based residential services for mentally handicapped people.* King Edward's Hospital Fund for London.

McConkey, R., Naughton, M. & Nugent, U. (1983). Have we met? Community contacts of adults who are mentally handicapped. *Mental Handicap.* 11(2), 57–9.

MIND (1982). *Getting together, sexual and social expression for mentally handicapped people.* MIND, London.

Quest for Improvement Limited, Slough (1992). *Pack of training material on personal relationships.* (In preparation).

Rose, J. & Holmes, S. (1991). Changing staff attitudes to the sexuality of people with mental handicaps. *Mental Handicap Research.* 4(1).

Stevens, S., Evered, C., O'Brien, R. & Wallace, E. (1988). Sex education: Who needs it? *Mental Handicap.* 16(4), 171–4.

Tyne, A. (1981). *The principle of normalisation: a foundation for effective services.* CMH Publications, London.

Williams, T., Tyson, J. & Keleher, R. (1989). Using mealtimes to develop interpersonal social skills in people with severe mental handicaps. *Mental Handicap.* 17(2), 74–7.

Wolfensberger, W. (1972). *The principle of normalisation in human services.* National Institute of Mental Retardation, Toronto.

Chapter 6

Integrated leisure opportunities

Steven Rose

People with learning difficulties have previously been denied the opportunity to integrate into mainstream daily living activities. The reasons for this denial are twofold: first, individuals with a learning difficulty have often lived in segregated settings; consequently opportunities for integration have been limited. Secondly, they have often been viewed as incapable of integration into mainstream activity due to an actual or perceived deficit in skills.

In fact, there are plenty of examples of individuals with severe learning difficulties and multiple disabilities being successfully integrated into challenging mainstream activities. Barton (1990) reported on a group which included people with learning difficulties who climbed Mount Kilimanjaro, Africa's highest mountain at 20 000 feet. Walker & Edinger (1988) provide an account of a child who has severe learning difficulties and physical disabilities being successfully integrated into an American summer camp. Rose (in press), reports on an autistic individual with severe learning difficulties who is taking part in a climb of the hazardous slopes of Mont Blanc, Europe's highest mountain.

This chapter examines the importance of leisure to all individuals, and examines the importance of integrated leisure opportunities for individuals who have a learning difficulty, and the possible reasons for the lack of integrated opportunities. Finally, drawing from the experiences of those who have successfully set up integrated leisure opportunities, strategies for integration are examined. The final part of the chapter is intended to be suitable for use as a checklist, by support workers working with an individual with a learning difficulty, as an aid to achieving integrated leisure opportunities.

In spite of the various beneficial changes to services for people with learning difficulties which have taken place over the past two decades (see Chapter 1), examples of true integration into mainstream leisure activities remain scarce. The relationships which are formed during recreational and leisure activities are fundamental to the quality of an individual's life (see Chapter 5). Non-parental relationships commence when the young person is first exposed to other people, which is usually at an early stage in development (Lewis & Rosenblum 1979), at playschool, junior school or before. The relationships which the person forms have a strong influence on all aspects of life, including with whom individuals choose to spend their leisure time and how they spend it; where they go on holiday; and often whom they marry or with whom they choose to share their life. Hence, it may be seen that the relationships formed play a major part in influencing the overall life direction of the person.

Leisure is an area of extreme importance in the lives of all individuals, since it provides opportunities to form, sustain or change relationships. Wade & Hoover (1985) describe two types of constraints on leisure opportunities in the lives of people with learning difficulties: external and internal constraints. External constraints include institutionalisation and social attitudes, while internal constraints may include such factors as physical fitness, motor skill deficits and lack of cognitive skills.

However, properly planned and supported programmes of recreation can assist the disabled individual to overcome external and internal constraints (Richardson 1986; Gold 1989; Rose 1990). In fact, the level of relationships enjoyed by individuals with disabilities can be seen as a measure of real acceptance into communities (Lutfiyya 1988). Furthermore, participation in leisure activities by disabled people has frequently been reported as producing beneficial changes in the attitudes of others towards them (Hamilton & Anderson 1983) and improvements to their self-esteem (Robbins 1991).

The leisure needs of people with learning difficulties are not being met to the same degree as those of non-disabled individuals. The reasons for this are varied and include poverty (Sylvester 1987) and segregation (Worth 1988). The more recent developments in community living do not automatically guarantee integration within the local community either (see Chapter 5) (Bratt & Johnson 1988). People with learning difficulties have been denied the experiences and activities that make it possible to make and keep friends. Limited contact with people in integrated settings has restricted the ability of individuals to develop their recreational and leisure interests, desires, likes, dislikes and talents. Additionally, the social isolation of people with learning difficulties has increased the individual's handicaps due to the fact that non-disabled people have not got to know and appreciate individuals with disabilities.

The desire to be with another person in a particular leisure activity has been identified as the most important aspect of leisure to the majority of people (Gunn 1982). There is also evidence which supports the idea that association and relationships with other people is an important aspect of leisure activities. In a study of 220 people, over 93 per cent of those studied stated that being with another person was one of the five most important aspects of their leisure experiences (Gunn 1982, p. 20).

The exclusion from mainstream leisure activities is, for many individuals with learning difficulties, a deep-rooted and ongoing problem, the effects of which have been built up over many years. Many individuals have cherished memories associated with leisure experiences which start in early childhood. Such memories might include early childhood games with one or both parents; building sandcastles on the beach; helping in the garden; going camping with the scouts/guides; playing team games such as hockey or football, or entertaining friends for the first time in a new home.

All of these memories are based on leisure experiences and most involve relationships with other people; they can never be replaced, and they stay with the individual for life. These sorts of experience are considered commonplace and everyday by most people, and are often taken for granted. However, such experiences are often missing from the lives of those with learning difficulties. The individual with a learning difficulty, who has grown up without the opportunity to acquire these cherished memories of leisure activities and make relationships, would seem to be at a significant disadvantage.

However, in practice much can be done to redress the balance, and most individuals soon respond to the opportunity to mix with others and form relationships. The integration of individuals with severe disabilities into mainstream leisure activities is seldom straightforward. The individual's fitness and levels of motor and cognitive skills need to be taken into account, together with the environment of integration, and an individualised strategy and support package needs to be worked out. The approach needs to be considered in three stages, which are planning, intervention and maintenance.

From the outset it must be appreciated that the benefits of integrated leisure activities for individuals with severe learning difficulties far outweigh those of segregated activities (Rose 1990). These benefits include:

- Providing opportunities to form, sustain or change relationships.

- Can be seen as a measure of real acceptance into community.

- Beneficial changes in the attitudes of others towards the individual with a disability.

- The opportunity to make and keep friends.

- The opportunity to be with another person.

The remainder of this chapter describes some of the evaluative work on integrated activities which has taken place, examines strategies for

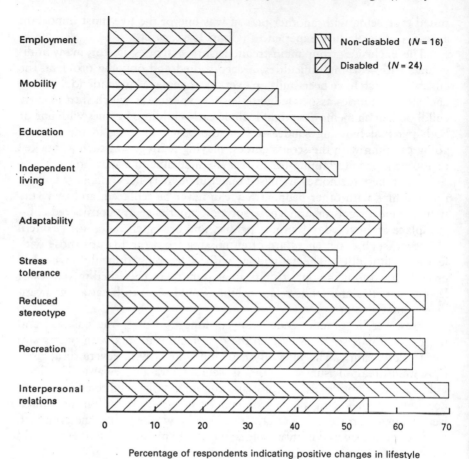

Figure 6.1 Summary of results from integrated wilderness adventure: effects on personal lifestyle traits on persons with and without disabilities (McAvoy *et al.* 1989).

integrating individuals with severe disabilities into mainstream leisure activities, and offers some practical advice based on successful attempts at setting up integrated leisure activities for individuals with severe disabilities.

The beneficial effects of integrated recreation programmes to individuals with and without disabilities have been identified (McAvoy & Schleien 1988), together with the effects of community-based programmes (Schleien & Meyer 1988). McAvoy *et al.* (1989) studied the effects of participation in Wilderness Inquiry adventures on the personal and lifestyle traits of persons with and without disabilities. A total of 40 people (24 with disabilities and 16 without disabilities) were studied using both quantitative and qualitative methods. The results (Figure 6.1) indicated that participation in wilderness adventures can lead to positive attitude and lifestyle changes for those with and without disabilities. Positive changes included attitudes towards persons of varying abilities, interpersonal relationships, confidence levels, willingness to take risks, feelings about self, goal-setting abilities, tolerance of stress and increased capability to approach new situations.

Walker & Edinger (1988) identified the following as some of the key elements to a successful activity, involving the integration of a child with severe physical disabilities and learning difficulties in a summer camp:

- Individualised support.

- A well-thought-out and financed programme.

- The recognition of the need of children with disabilities to participate and react with non-disabled friends.

- Small-scale integrational attempts.

When these strategies were adopted the most severely disabled child was integrated into mainstream leisure and daily living activities. Individually planned and delivered support is the fundamental ingredient to successful integration (Walker 1990). Non-disabled children and helpers can also benefit from integrational experiences (Schleien *et al.* 1985). Rynders *et al.* (1990) evaluated a two-week integrated camping experience, which involved three children with severe physical disabilities and learning difficulties. They found that the children demonstrated substantially improved skills in targeted activities, and that children with and without disabilities increased their attempts to make social contacts with each other. The findings indicated that there were more ratings reflective of friendship, and that there were increased positive perceptions among staff of the benefits of the integrated camp.

Wilderness Inquiry, based in Minneapolis, Minnesota, is an organisation which sets out to bring together people with and without disabilities, and to promote growth and understanding through wilderness experiences. The belief is that shared adventure is one of the most effective ways to facilitate social integration and personal growth amongst diverse groups of people. Its mission is 'to provide active outdoor adventure opportunities that integrate people with and without disabilities in experiences which inspire personal growth, develop peer relationships, and enhance awareness of the environment'.

Wilderness Inquiry was established in 1978 to allow people of all abilities to share the benefits and adventure of wilderness travel. It first attracted publicity a year later (Corty 1979). Since then, Wilderness Inquiry has run integrated adventure activities on a worldwide basis in such areas as the Rocky Mountains, the North American and Canadian Wildernesses, Australia, the USSR and the Arctic, and these have been widely reported

(Hevesi 1987; Crawford 1989; Lias 1989; Peterson 1989; Chanco 1990; Ernst 1990; Lindler 1990; Simmons 1990; Watson 1990). It is non-profit making, and has over the years allowed thousands of people access to some of the most beautiful and remote parts of the world. Most of the activities of Wilderness Inquiry are undertaken on water or snow, thus using canoes or dog sleds to ameliorate the effects of physical disabilities.

Drawing upon the lessons from the above evaluative work, other relevant evaluations (Ray *et al.* 1986, Certo *et al.* 1983, Schleien & Ray 1988) and the personal experience of the author, it is possible to identify a five-point strategy for successful integration. This strategy is presented below in the form of a checklist, which represents the common elements repeatedly identified in successful integration programmes.

■ Strategies for integration

1. Individualised support
On each occasion when an individual is integrated into a mainstream leisure activity, the support requirements must be identified. The support requirements of an individual may be described as the extra resources required to ameliorate the handicapping effects of the disability in the environment in question. The environment could be a rugby club, scouts, dancing classes or a luncheon club for elderly persons. The individualised support requirements of the client will need to be tailored specifically to the support requirements of the client in that particular environment.

No two individual support requirements are likely to be exactly the same, and nor will the integrational environment, e.g. one club may have disabled access whilst another may not, or the age group or social background of members may be entirely different in two separate dancing classes. Therefore the strategy for integration which worked in the first dancing class may not be applicable in the second.

It is also important to recognise that there will be ongoing support needs, which may fluctuate. Most programmes with people with learning difficulties encourage moves towards independence, the implication being gradually reduced levels of support. However, when integrating individuals into mainstream leisure activities it is important that support is flexible enough to respond to the need for increased support. Increased support requirements can be brought about by internal changes, e.g. decreased confidence or poor health, or external changes, e.g. altered club rules or changed timetable.

Whilst with careful preparation most individuals and organisations will welcome people with disabilities, few will be enthusiastic about taking on personal care needs, such as feeding or assistance with toileting. These are not leisure activities, and participation in the leisure activity in question will have been the motivating factor for the other people attending. Many well-intentioned integrational attempts fail because assumptions are made that members of the public will be willing to become involved in supporting the personal care needs of the disabled individual.

2. Strategies for funding

Integrating individuals with learning difficulties into mainstream leisure activities usually requires extra money. The reasons for the extra costs include transport, entry fees, appropriate leisure clothing and equipment, volunteer expenses and cost of support staff. Any attempt at setting up an integrated leisure experience which does not identify and plan for the extra costs will fail. An individual strategy to meet these costs will need to be identified. Nowadays, support staff in both the statutory and independent sectors find themselves working in cash-limited services, probably to a fairly tight contractual arrangement. In these situations the prospect of identifying extra funds will seem daunting.

It is possible that a support agency will have funds to meet these types of activity, or that individuals can afford to fund the activity themselves, though often this will not be the case. The funding requirements will vary depending on the individual support needs, which will vary according to the level of disability and the complexity and ambition of the leisure activity.

3. Extra staff and transportation

The creation of integrated leisure activities is likely to create extra staffing requirements. The extra staffing input may be in support of the individuals participating in the integrated leisure activity, or to cover the absence of the support staff from the normal workplace, such as a day centre or housing service. The extra staffing need must be clearly identified from the outset, and strategies to meet the requirement developed. Extra staff equates to extra money, and nowadays the prospect of securing additional resources is a remote one. However, if this problem is allowed to become a blockage then little progress will be made. This is the time to adopt the old adage 'there is no such thing as a problem, only solutions'.

It may well be that if the support worker is employed by a statutory or voluntary agency that some extra funds do exist, or that there is a special budget. It is definitely worth asking, although the answer may be disappointing. It is also possible that as the NHS and Community Care Act (Department of Health 1990) is implemented and the process of care management is developed, there may be enough flexibility to divert funds to support an innovative needs-led project. If the individual has a case or care manager, then they will need to be supported in requesting that their funding is allocated to this project.

There is less resistance in statutory services to the principle of using volunteers than there was a decade ago. The term volunteer in itself is not a helpful one, as it conjures up a picture of need and benevolence. There are local and national schemes, such as One to One, that provide people prepared to support an individual on a voluntary basis in leisure and other activities. An alternative and often more effective approach is to contact directly the club, society or recreation centre where the proposed activity is to take place, and attempt to find one or more individuals prepared to help out. This approach obviously needs careful planning, with a delicate balance to be struck between giving information to potential helpers and the individuals' personal privacy. In 1990 the author linked up a Venture Scout Unit with a small group of individuals with severe learning difficulties. The preparation took many hours over a number of months, and entailed accompanying them on a number of activities, including a weekend on Dartmoor. Now the individuals with learning difficulties regularly attend the Venture Scout activities with no support at all from the author. The use of voluntary support may still mean some extra expense; for instance it is usual to pay travelling expenses. As previously stated, an assumption that a volunteer will also be prepared to deal with personal care needs is likely to lead to failed integrational attempts.

Other options include the creative re-structuring of staffing rotas, and vacancies can aid the situation. For example, it may be possible to change one full-time post to three part-time posts. If an individual is being supported to attend a swimming club, or other similar club or activity, and there are scarce staffing/support resources, then initially attending underused sessions can be advantageous. In such a situation more support may be available from instructors, and in a more relaxed setting others may be more willing to become involved.

Finally, plan any transport requirements for the individual, volunteers, support workers and equipment. The integrating of the individual will be less likely to be successful if they arrive late or have to leave early due to constraints of transport arrangements or staff rotas.

4. 'More' does not mean better
Attempts at setting up integrated leisure activities can be successful in the early days, thus enthusing volunteers, support workers and members of the public. A common reaction to this from the host organisation, after an individual has successfully been integrated, is to offer to have more people with disabilities involved in their activities. It is easy to get carried along by the wave of enthusiasm and to introduce more individuals with disabilities to the activity. If this does become the case it will become a self-defeating exercise. When a successful activity has been established, it should be evaluated and the key reasons for its success drawn out, so that the strategy can be used elsewhere with other individuals.

5. Know the 'culture'
Attempts to integrate individuals into mainstream activities can fail if the

people supporting them fail to understand fully the culture of the organisation. For example, if part of the current children's culture is 'Mutant Turtles', and a nine-year-old with learning difficulties is taken to an activity wearing a 'Ghostbusters' T-shirt, he or she is highly likely to be rejected. In this instance the learning difficulty becomes a secondary factor to the rejection, with the out-of-vogue T-shirt likely to be the primary factor causing the child to be singled out. Another example would be if a young man wished to join a local rugby club; he would be at a double disadvantage if the support worker was unfamiliar with the rules, culture and game of rugby. Such clubs are often most willing to accept an individual with a learning difficulty into their midst. However, one must be prepared to join in the after-match antics, and again the attempt is likely to fail if the support worker is a teetotaller! Finally, it is important that those embarking upon setting up integrated leisure activities have clearly defined criteria for success from the outset. It is not possible to prescribe criteria for success in these guidelines. The needs and requirements of individuals will vary and there are numerous different leisure experiences to consider. A true measure of integration must be developed on each occasion. For example, if an individual goes to the local public house with a support worker twice a week this does not amount to integration. However, if the individual goes to the public house twice a week, is welcomed by regular customers, participates in conversations and other activities, and has her or his own tankard behind the bar, then a measure of integration has been achieved.

■ Conclusion

The benefits of participating in integrated leisure activities have been well documented (Rose 1990; McAvoy & Schleien 1988; Schleien & Meyer 1988; McAvoy *et al.* 1989). These beneficial effects, which are in keeping with O'Brien's accomplishments (see Chapter 8), are thought to include increased competence, self esteem and ability to form and sustain relationships.

Whilst research indicates the benefits to clients from integrated leisure activities it should be remembered that these activities are enjoyable in their own right. Consequently they should not be viewed as being purely therapeutic activities. After all, many people spend their leisure time undertaking activities which they enjoy. This should also be the norm for people with a learning difficulty.

It is acknowledged that it may be difficult for staff to initiate integrated leisure activities. However, the use of the checklist provided would assist in this development. The key to successful integration is enthusiastic and motivated staff who also have an interest in the activity.

■ References

Barton, J. (1990). Conquerors in the African challenge. *Special Report, Bucks Herald,* 8 March.

Bratt, A. & Johnson, R. (1988). Changes in life style for young adults with profound handicaps following discharge from hospital care into a 'second generation' housing project. *Mental Handicap Research.* 1(1), 49–74.

Chanco, B. (1990). Great outdoors puts everyone on the same level. *Pioneer Press, AM Edition* (St Paul MN). 5 July.

Corty, J. (1979). Disabled blaze new trail in the wilds. *New York Times. Section 10.* 21 October.

Certo, N. J., Schleien, S. J. & Hunter, D. (1983). An ecological assessment inventory to facilitate community recreation participation by severely disabled individuals. *Therapeutic Recreation Journal.* 17(3), 29–38.

Crawford, R. (1989). Brothers of one fate. *Sailor: Minnesota Suburban Newspapers.* 6 September.

Department of Health (1990). *NHS and Community Care Act 1990.* HMSO, London.

Ernst, K. (1990). A new sense of freedom. *Wilderness,* 53(188), 39–43.

Gold, D. (1989). *Ten commonly asked questions about recreation and integration. The pursuit of leisure: enriching the lives of people who have a disability* (rev. edn). The G. Allan Roeher Institute, York University, Ontario.

Gunn, S. L. (1982). Value of relationships in leisure. *Journal of Leisurability.* 9(2).

Hamilton, M. A. & Anderson, S. C. (1983). Effects of leisure activities on attitudes toward people with disabilities. *Therapeutic Recreation Journal.* 17(3).

Hevesi, D. (1987). A sense of adventure and then some. *New York Times.* 5 July.

Lewis, M. & Rosenblum, L. A. (eds) (1979). *The child and its family.* Plenum, New York.

Lias, G. (1989). Wilderness inquiry: Integration through adventure. *Impact.* 2(3), 2.

Lindler, B. (1990). Outdoors: Wheelchairs, wilderness and water. *Great Falls Tribune* (Minnesota). 6 September.

Lutfiyya, Z. M. (1988). Other than clients: reflections on relationships between people with disabilities and typical people. *Tash Newsletter.* September, 3–5.

McAvoy, L. & Schleien, S. J. (1988). Effects of integrated interpretive programs on persons with and without disabilities. *National Association of Interpretation Research.* 4(2), 13–26.

McAvoy, L., Schatz, E., Stutz, M., Schleien, S. J. & Lias, G. (1989). Integrated wilderness adventure: Effects on personal and lifestyle traits of persons with and without disabilities. *Therapeutic Recreation Journal.* 23(3), 50–64.

Peterson, B. (1989). Citizen diplomats: Kayaking to friendship in the Soviet Union. *Sunday Magazine: Star Tribune* (Minneapolis). 15 October.

Ray, M. T., Schleien, S., Larson, A., Rutten, T. & Slick, C. (1986). Integrating persons with disabilities into community leisure environments. *Journal of Expanding Horizons in Therapeutic Recreation.* 1(1), 49–55.

Richardson. D. (1986). Outdoor adventure: Wilderness programs for the physically disabled. *Parks and Recreation.* 21(11), 43–5.

Robbins, M. (1991). Sweet Challenge. *Nursing Times*, 87(1).

Rose, S. (1990). The value of outdoor activities. *Nursing*. 4(21), 12–16.

Rose, S. (in press). An exploratory investigation into the benefits of adventurous outdoor activities to individuals with severe learning difficulties. *Mental Handicap Research*.

Rynders, J., Schleien, S. J. & Mustonen, T. (1990). Integrating children with severe disabilities for intensified outdoor education: focus on feasibility. *Mental Retardation*. 128(1), 7–14.

Schleien, S. & Ray, M. T. (1988). *Community recreation and persons with disabilities: Strategies for integration*. Paul H. Brookes Publishing Co., Baltimore.

Schleien, S. J. & Meyer, L. H. (1988). Community based recreation programs for persons with severe developmental disabilities. In *Expanding systems of service delivery for persons with developmental disabilities* (ed M. Powers). pp. 93–122. Paul H. Brookes Publishing Co., Baltimore.

Schleien, S. J., Olson, K., Rogers, N. & McLafferty, M. (1985). Integrating children with severe handicaps into recreation and physical education programs. *Journal of Park and Recreation Administration*. 3(1), 50–66.

Simmons, C. (1990). Wilderness Inquiry. *Abilities*. 1(4), 3.

Sylvester, C. (1987). The politics of leisure, freedom and poverty. *Parks and Recreation Magazine*. American National Recreation and Parks Association, January.

Wade, G. M., & Hoover, J. H. (1985). Mental retardation as a constraint on leisure. In *Constraints on leisure* (eds M. G. Wade & C. C. Thomas). Springfield, Illinois.

Walker, P. (1990). *Supports for children and teens with severe disabilities in integrated recreation/leisure activities*. Center on Human Policy, Syracuse University, New York.

Walker, P. & Edinger, B. (1988). The kid from cabin 17. *Camping Magazine*. May, 18–21.

Watson, C. (1990). Wilderness Inquiry provides real adventure for everybody. *Star Tribune* (Minneapolis). 4 February.

Worth, P. (1988). You've got a friend. *The Pursuit of Leisure: Enriching lives with people who have a disability*. The G. Allan Roeher Institute, Toronto.

Chapter 7

Psychotherapeutic approaches with people with learning difficulties

Tony Taylor

■ Introduction

The use of psychotherapy with clients with learning difficulties is a relatively recent development which has occurred over the past ten years. The first publication in relation to using this approach with this client group was in 1981. Following this much work has been undertaken by the Tavistock Clinic. In addition to this a number of people have become interested in the use of psychotherapy with people with learning difficulties (Cole 1989; Marler & Carroll-Williams 1989; Humphreys *et al.* 1990). As people with learning difficulties strive to reach their maximum potential they will increasingly need access to the full range of therapies which is available to everyone in the population. This could lead to an increase in demand for this type of service. This chapter will explore some models of psychotherapeutic intervention and will consider a case study in detail to indicate the practical applicability of psychotherapy. The case study presented is a young person with mild learning difficulties. As yet much of the psychotherapeutic work is carried out with people with mild and moderate learning difficulties. However, as therapists become more skilled it may be possible to use this intervention with clients with severe learning difficulties.

■ Psychotherapy

Psychotherapy has been defined as the systematic use of a relationship between therapist and client which produces changes in cognition, behaviour and feelings (Holmes & Lindley 1990). Therapeutic outcomes for the client are the ability to form satisfying relationships, personal independence and emotional freedom. According to Frank (1974), psychotherapy is offered or sought when a person's disability or suffering appears to have a significant psychological or emotional component. The *Observer* newspaper (1988) provided an illustration of this where two men and three women were asked why they had entered long-term individual therapy. The answers given ranged from experiencing nightmares to being unhappy for years. According to Bloch (1981), individual psychotherapy takes one of eight forms. These psychotherapies are distinguished from one another by their goals, techniques and target of intervention. They all have the common aim of instilling in the client the sense that they can attain a measure of self control, have a reasonable self-image and have a sense that they are capable (Bloch 1982). This is in opposition to the belief commonly held by the client that they are the victim of the environment. Another common feature of the varying types of psychotherapies is the interpersonal experiences of the client and therapist. These experiences, when therapeutic, may be classed as success experiences which enable the demoralised individual to gain or regain positive self-esteem (Bloch 1981; Frank 1974). This in turn equips the individual to gain control over those aspects of his or her life which are causing concern, to the extent that the disturbing symptoms will be reduced or eliminated (Rutter 1982). External factors need to be taken into account in the reduction of symptoms (Sinason 1989) and an illustration is provided later which includes this aspect of therapy.

Supportive psychotherapy is the simplest and most widely used form of interpersonal therapy (McKenna 1990). This is generally termed counselling (Pedder 1989), and is considered as level 1 psychotherapy. Level 2 psychotherapy is formal and its use requires the use of a theoretical rationale (Rowan 1983). It is what the most effective professionals do. Level 3 dynamic psychotherapy is a specialist level of intervention (Pedder 1989).

□ Supportive psychotherapy

Supportive psychotherapy can be defined as the form of treatment which a therapist offers to clients in order to sustain them when they are unable to manage their lives independently (Bloch 1981). The principal aims of treatment are the promotion of the clients' greatest possible psychological and social functioning by restoring and reinforcing their abilities to manage their lives and to increase their self-confidence and self-esteem.

The components of therapy are reassurance, explanation, guidance, suggestion, encouragement, effecting changes in the client's environment and permission for catharsis (release of pent-up feelings). Whilst this model (Bloch 1981) has as its aim the treatment of the individual it is adaptable to therapeutic group work. The components are similar to Yalom's (1985) therapeutic factors which operate in therapy groups.

Dependency on the therapist is a danger where an individual's inability to cope may be enduring (Bloch 1981). To avoid this it is necessary to transfer the support provided by the therapist to members of the individual's family, friends or other carers, provided that they have the necessary skills and abilities to take on this role. The timing of this transference will be identified jointly by the client and therapist, the latter having previously discussed the strategy of withdrawal with a supervisor.

The application of these strategies, whether individually or in groups, will occur in the context of the therapist and client relationship and in a therapeutic environment.

□ Supportive/analytic psychotherapy

Bloch's (1981) model of psychotherapy can be adapted to include psychoanalytic concepts, such as those of the unconscious, transference and interpretation (Rycroft 1968). Unconscious conflicts may be made comprehensible to the client by the use of interpretation and transference. In transference the client tends to transfer to the therapist attitudes about important figures in her or his life (Frank 1974). Interpretation may be made to foster the therapeutic alliance, or used only in supervision sessions to enable the therapist to understand affective interactions between the therapist and client. This amalgamation of 'forms' of psychotherapy may be termed supportive/analytic psychotherapy.

□ Psychotherapy and people with learning difficulties

Emotional disturbance in individuals with a mild learning difficulty is intimately connected with their intellectual failures. This has been termed handicap awareness (Grunewald 1983). They are frequently aware of being stigmatised (Szivos & Griffiths 1990), which adds to the burden of handicap (Sinason 1989), and this may cause individuals to become discouraged and demoralised, which further reduces their ability to function (Frank 1974). These difficulties are often further compounded by an inability to communicate effectively. These factors may cause the individual to become aggressive, withdrawn, neurotic or psychotic (Grunewald 1983).

Psychotherapy may be of assistance by enabling clients to make stress-reducing changes in their lives and to take a more optimistic view of the future (Frank 1974). This view should engender hope for the fulfilment of the individual's need for recognition, affection and sense of competence (Bloch 1981). Previously the satisfaction of these needs has been impeded by the emotion, attitude and behaviour of the individual, which have arisen out of a defective emotional development (Grunewald 1983). Brandon (1989) indicates that the use of behavioural techniques has been the dominant therapeutic intervention utilised with people with learning difficulties. Brandon (1989) states that by utilising this approach behaviourally challenging people have been treated by a process that ignores the individual's psychological and physical well-being and denies the context of the behaviour. Rarely do professionals ask 'why are these people angry?' While the domination of behaviourism has lasted three decades, two antithetical influences have come into the ascendancy in services. These are normalisation (see Chapter 1) and psychoanalytic psychotherapy. Normalisation ensures that the context of the person's behaviour is defined by focusing attention on what people with learning difficulties can achieve, and how service systems should be designed to maximise that achievement (Gardner & O'Brien 1990).

Psychotherapy addresses the issue of emotional well-being. Practitioners of psychoanalytical psychotherapy will ask the question or investigate 'Why are you angry?', and eventually offer an explanation to the client and/or carers, with the client's permission.

■ The use of psychotherapy in practice: Erik's story

□ History

When Erik's parents could no longer contend with his severe epilepsy, he was admitted to a special boarding school for children with learning difficulties. He was eight years old at this time. At the age of 16 he left school and went to live in a hospital unit near his home. It was during this time that Erik's violent and disruptive behaviour, which had commenced at school, became more intense and frequent. This episodic violence, which was frequently managed by the use of forcible restraint and sedation, deteriorated to the extent that eventually he was transferred to a large hospital, 30 miles away from home. He lived at the hospital for several years during which time he formed a relationship with a young woman who became his girlfriend, and worked regularly in the hospital grounds as an assistant gardner.

In 1988, Botley House, a secure unit for behaviourally challenging young people, opened in Erik's home town. He was duly transferred to the new facility, and was one of eight residents. He was, by this time, 26 years old. Erik was soon found a job as an assistant to the estate workers in the local hospital. He held this job for a while until taunts from one particular worker caused him to lose his temper. Following this he was sacked. Erik later revealed that on the day he was sacked he had also been taunted at home. Being taunted both at home and later at work proved intolerable and he hurled abuse at his tormentors and slammed a door. This behaviour had the consequence of Erik losing his employment.

□ Family relationships

Erik's parents had divorced ten years previously; coincidentally, during this time Erik's violence at the first hospital unit had intensified. This may be attributed to Erik's perception that he was being abandoned for a second time, the first abandonment being when he was admitted to a residential school. It was not known by anyone whether the divorce was brought about by the cost (Corney 1986) of caring for a child who has a learning difficulty and epilepsy, but Erik somehow 'knew' that his placing intolerable demands on them, 'through having fits which caused commotion', must have brought about the split. His guilt about this caused him to be full of self-hatred. His inability to blame them for their 'cruelty' in not caring for him was the pivot of his ambivalence towards them. The objectification of this loving/rejecting ambivalence between parents and child was Erik's teddy bear, treasured through childhood and adolescence and called Mr Nobody.

Throughout his stay in residential units, Erik had visited or been visited by his parents on alternate weekends, a pattern which rarely deviated. After the divorce, he would see his mother one weekend and his father the next. More recently, either parent might take him to see his younger brother and his wife. Any deviation from this routine was strongly resisted by Erik, to the extent of passing up the opportunity of extra visits which might be offered on special occasions, such as birthdays.

Erik's relationship with his parents can be characterised by guilt for not being born perfect, resentment and ambivalence. His relationship to his brother, his only sibling, is deeply coloured by envy, for his brother not only 'dethroned' him (Orgler 1973), but had actually taken his place, confirmed upon his being sent away to a special school while his brother remained at home. During therapy Erik graphically told of his feelings towards his brother.

□ The initial interview

Erik's story was one of recent multiple losses, his reaction to which had become more than usually violent and disruptive according to his key-worker, who was a member of the house staff with particular responsibility for assisting Erik. It was the key-worker who made the referral for psychotherapy.

Erik himself spoke of the loss of his job, about which he was still angry (albeit that it happened five months ago), and of the fact that he still missed his girlfriend, and had found no other. The staff had not assisted Erik in maintaining the relationship after the transfer, and he now faced the imminent departure of his key-worker, the third such departure since he had arrived at the unit. It was known to Erik that the staff member was leaving to gain promotion, as had the others, but despite this reality, someone had told him, or he had told himself, that he was driving people away with his demands. As he had 'split' his parents, so he was now splitting the staff group. The therapist also learned that he was receiving once-weekly individual art therapy, and a once-weekly hydrotherapy session. He had suffered a mild hemiplegia, causing his now atrophied right arm to be flexed to his body. His other current treatment was tranquillising medication and anti-convulsant medication, supervised by a consultant psychiatrist.

The psychotherapist offered to see Erik for one hour a week to give him the opportunity to talk privately and uninterruptedly about his relationships, which is something not possible within the unit. It was explained to Erik that he could meet the psychotherapist five or six times at the same hour on the same day, after which he could say whether he wished to continue. Erik agreed to this arrangement, and a date was set for the first meeting. It was also agreed that he could make his own way to the therapy room, inform the therapist if he could not attend by telephoning the office, arrive on time and leave on time. The initial interview was concluded by the therapist walking with him to the therapy room, which was situated in the day service centre some five hundred yards from his home. The centre provides occupation and recreational activities to people in the community and those residing in residential units.

□ **Life in Botley House**

Of the eight residents in Botley House, Erik and his friend Gerald were the most capable, both making full use of speech and being able to perform all basic self-help functions, such as feeding, washing and dressing. The other six residents, Erik explained, 'didn't understand', that is they did not speak in sentences, and did little to help themselves. He referred to them by using some characteristic behaviour to identify them. 'The trouble with Ann is she steals food', and 'The trouble with Tom is he runs off down the road', both causing upset within the unit. This account was given in an early session. He made it clear, also early in the sessions, that there were frequent episodes of violence within the unit. Sometimes he was an instigator/participant and sometimes not. Another individual, often cited, who would be at the centre of these incidents was Andrew. The following extract illustrates this.

> Something happened on Sunday. I was not involved. The staff sent
> me to another unit to get a break from it. I had my lunch there.
> After the incident was over I returned to the house and slept. There
> was another incident yesterday. Andrew kept banging the windows
> with his fist. I was getting shaved at the time, until one broke. It was
> an accident but he cut his hand and there was blood everywhere.
> Like a murder film. On Sunday things were out of control. I was
> frightened.

Two weeks after this report, the session started with Erik hurtling into the room, and throwing himself into the chair. Very loudly and angrily he stated that there had been a bad start to the day. Breakfast was late, because staff had had to deal with Andrew. 'The trouble with Andrew is he doesn't understand.' Erik became so angry that he left the dining room, went upstairs to his room and hit the wardrobe, breaking the door. These incidents were commonplace. Erik was never sure if staff did all they could to keep things under control. It seemed clear from the regularity of reports concerning Andrew that he was a suitable object into whom Erik could project his aggressive parts (Salzberger-Wittenberg 1970). It often happened that an episode would be brought under control with staff physically restraining Erik by using a handling procedure. The last stage of this procedure allowed for the administration of a tranquillising injection. Erik reported that he felt damaged after such episodes. He hated the idea of featuring on an incident report, though he frequently did.

The routine which these episodes interrupted was described in the sessions as 'Hydrotherapy on Mondays, and Tuesdays I come here, Wednesdays I have Art Therapy, nothing particular on Thursdays or Fridays'. Occasionally, to earn a little more money Erik would wash the staff members' cars, though such opportunities were limited. He would listen to his country and western tapes, watch television and walk to the town centre for some minor purchase. One of the out-buildings had been given over to Erik as a woodwork room, and some time was spent there, but this was dependent to a large extent on a member of staff working with him and this was often not possible. 'You're not the only one living here', he would mimic the staff.

During the day his friend Gerald attended the local day service unit, and all the other residents spent at least part of the day in outside activities. This meant that Erik was left on his own for much of the day and he often slept through boredom at these times. He bitterly resented the gardeners who had caused him to lose his job. His loss of status plus his drop in income, and the lack of structure to the day, all caused him problems which would only be resolved by getting another job, a prospect not in view for the foreseeable future. Since he could not go looking for a job on his own, he was powerless to bring about change in this area.

☐ **The 26th session**

The psychotherapist had arrived as usual ten minutes before the start of the session. After a while Erik's enraged voice could be heard, as he stormed down the corridor to the room. He kicked the wedge from under the door, which closes it, entered the room and threw himself into the chair. He repeated what had been said by him before he entered the room 'Big mouth. I was okay until she [Sally, a staff member], opened her big mouth'. She had asked him if he was going to arrange for the repair of his electric razor, which because it was broken had been kept in the office desk drawer. 'Getting it fixed is not so easy. Anyway, I wet-shave now and she was the one who taught me.' He still shouted, he was very angry. The psychotherapist asked him who had given him the razor. His father had given it to him, he said, but it had previously belonged to his brother who had discarded it. He had broken it accidentally (Freud 1934) by dropping it, and could not afford to have it repaired as he had no job. Also it was getting near Christmas, so the repair shop would take longer to repair it. It was best to leave it for some other time, to forget it. He shouted louder still, 'Sometimes I get jealous! I am the older brother. It's usual for the older brother to give things to the younger one. He's married and drives a car. I have fits!' He screamed, 'Look at this hand' he held up his atrophied right hand. Tears came to his eyes, he slumped back into the chair, and asked despairingly 'Why was I born like it?'.

The psychotherapist had intuitively supposed the origins of the razor to be the key to Erik's distress. Sally's question had been experienced as an attack; she had in a very real way, caught Erik unawares. What had been successfully repressed, his destructive envy towards his brother, had been brought partly back into consciousness by the question but not into full awareness, causing anger to be displaced on to Sally as he re-experienced the rage, and the acute guilt feelings connected with it, which he felt at the time of the gift. The question, 'Who gave you the razor?' had the effect of an interpretation, making fully conscious the forgotten conflict.

The psychotherapist said that he understood his having mixed feelings about the razor. He did not wish to use it for the injustices it symbolised, nor could he throw it away, as it might be evidence of love and concern from his father, so he had been pleased for it to be out of sight and out of mind. Erik now knew that dropping the razor had been an attack on his brother, and he had been relieved by the catharsis that had taken place as a result (Bloch 1981).

At the end of the session it was agreed that he would give himself two or three days to decide what to do about the razor. He left on time, calm and composed, having had a difficult, despairing, anxious part of himself held (Salzberger-Wittenberg 1970).

□ **The therapeutic alliance**

The episode cited illustrates several aspects of the relationship, at this point six months old. The therapy room was considered a safe place, in which anger, envy and frustration could be expressed. The relationship permitted painful feelings to be expressed (Bloch 1981), and the therapist acted as a container for the feelings in a way that the client understands. 'This person cares. He or she can bear to look at my despair without being afraid of it and seeking ways to avoid it. He or she is someone who can feel despair and not break down under it, and this gives me hope of despair being tolerable' (Salzberger-Wittenberg 1970). Erik had earlier sought and received assurance that it was okay to come to therapy if feeling angry or enraged. It is a time when a client needs most help, and an acute crisis gives the therapist an optimal point for therapeutic intervention, as the client is less defended and most anxious for help (Salzberger-Wittenberg 1970).

However disorganising the episode with the razor had been, Erik was still sufficiently organised to attend for therapy on time, and with the capacity for work. The rhythm of therapy had not been broken, or rather the relationship had withstood this external battering, being seen as a safe haven in an otherwise chaotic existence. Erik is certain of his hour. In six months he has turned up at the arranged time to find the psychotherapist waiting for him and eager to work. The therapists' display of eagerness and optimism (Bloch 1981) carries the client, who may arrive despondent and discouraged, an attitude which indicates that discussing problems may be a way of finding a solution (Salzberger-Wittenberg 1970). This display must be conveyed to the client without words, by a patient, thoughtful, alert disposition, allowing him, in his own time, to begin using his hour. In the razor episode the therapist spoke only three times during the entire session; otherwise communication was given by eye contact, body posture and guided by judiciously timed use of para-language, at other times maintaining an attitude of respectful serious attention (Bloch 1981). Erik left with an understanding of why he was so enraged, which had not been available to him prior to the session. Some mental order had been brought about by correct naming and identification of the feelings, anger and jealously, which then became more manageable instead of being vague and limitless (Salzberger-Wittenberg 1970). These understandings combined with Erik's idea that he can manage the demands of the relationship over a relatively long period of time instils a feeling of mastery over external and internal events not hitherto experienced, with a consequent increase in self-esteem, the necessary precursor for change. McKenna (1990) states that by experiencing a healthy relationship with the therapist the client could learn to have more satisfying relationships in general.

□ **King's Hill Centre – A step toward social relationships**

King's Hill Centre is a project for up to twelve young people with mild to moderate learning difficulties. The centre provides recreational activities, social skills training and assistance in using community facilities, such as shops, parks, libraries and sports facilities. It is open two days a week. The programme is run by volunteers, who have been recruited to the project by the community nurse for people with learning difficulties, who has overall responsibility for the project and acts as a coordinator. The centre users are nearly all under thirty, and most of them are under twenty-five. Like Erik, they have 'failed' in open employment, finished with employment training, or are waiting or not wanting to go to the local authority day services unit. They were all socially isolated individuals prior to attending the centre. Social contacts were enhanced by attending the centre in a protective type of setting where the user can derive pleasure from pursuits that are intrinsically enjoyable and worthwhile (Bloch 1981).

Erik had been referred to the centre prior to starting therapy by his psychiatrist, who saw the benefits of his attending as providing social contacts, a degree of structure to his week and supporting his efforts to find another job. The centre was within walking distance of Botley House. However, he fell short of meeting the criteria for admission on two counts: his epilepsy and his violent outbursts, neither of which, it was felt by the house staff, the volunteers would be able to deal with. Consequently the referral laid dormant for several months.

Two things had changed since the referral had been made, however. The community nurse, previously only paying occasional visits to the centre for relatively short periods of an hour or so, was now able to remain at the project throughout its opening hours. Secondly, Erik had entered therapy, attending regularly for three months, making his own way to the session and back, tolerating the demands of the hour's work to the extent that it seemed to the therapist appropriate to reconsider the possibility of attendance at the centre. Therapy was stress-reducing (Frank 1974), and could be geared to supporting Erik in his efforts to use the centre; that is work could have the aim of bringing about a change in his environment, which is an aim of supportive psychotherapy. The volunteers could be supported by the community nurse, who would be responsible for Erik while at the centre. At the end of the tenth session Erik was asked to consider the idea.

Over the next two weeks Erik organised his start at the centre, with advice and encouragement sought and given in his therapy sessions. The psychiatrist who had made the referral agreed the timing of the strategy, in supervisory sessions with the therapist. Erik apprised his key-worker and the other unit staff of his intentions. The community nurse visited the staff to give further information and carry arrangements forward. Erik's art therapist agreed to re-schedule his art therapy sessions so that he could attend on Wednesdays. The art therapist also proposed a visit to the centre, with a view of starting an art therapy group on Wednesday afternoons. If the group became established, Erik would have the option of terminating individual art therapy and moving over to the group. All involved had agreed to the proposed strategy of Erik's regular attendance at the centre. When all arrangements had been finalised, the community nurse arranged to escort Erik to the centre on his first two visits, after which Erik would attend the centre unaccompanied.

Over the next few sessions Erik talked enthusiastically about his visits to the centre. He liked the people who were there, and the activities he had been involved in. His new routine was discussed, and how things were changing for the better as far as daily occupation was concerned. At the beginning of therapy he had had three one hour activities scheduled. This had now been expanded to Monday and Wednesday at the centre, with psychotherapy on Tuesday and art therapy on Thursday. The hydrotherapy had ceased. Erik and the therapist were making progress in bringing about change, as predicted. This had been brought about by advice, guidance and encouragement, offered at the right moment in the sessions. Continuing support would now be necessary for Erik to make full use of the centre. How would he operate in a new peer group? There would need to be close cooperation of all professionals involved for the enterprise to succeed.

☐ **Client–therapist relationship**

The client–therapist relationship in supportive psychotherapy allows the therapist to be directive: the question asked is 'How can I help modify my client's impoverished social environment to his best advantage?' (Bloch 1981). Directing Erik to King's· Hill Centre was the beginning of a joint strategy to promote better psychological and social functioning and increase self-esteem, the two principal aims of supportive psychotherapy. Successful experiences were reported in the therapy sessions: 'I've been out every day this week. Got a kiss from Valerie [another centre user] last time I went to the centre, so yesterday I gave her one. I couldn't go round to her place though'. On walking into the room: 'Guess what I've been doing? Playing table tennis with Pat', or: 'Went to the centre yesterday and got a bit excited about Christmas coming. I did the washing up after lunch to work it off.' Therapist: 'You stayed in control then?' Erik: 'Yes.'

In the twenty sessions which followed Erik's start at King's Hill centre he mentioned attendance at the centre in nine sessions. As with the three examples already given, he talked of his success and received appropriate congratulatory responses. Where an issue needed exploring, such as 'Why do you feel you couldn't go round to Valerie's house?' it was with advice and explanation as necessary. In the third example above, which it was later learned from the community nurse needed his intervention, the exchange does not convey the nuances of the report. Erik's tone of voice conveyed embarrassment and regret, and the tone of the therapist's voice added the unspoken 'as we said, you would stay in control'.

In ten months at the centre Erik has not had an epileptic seizure and he has needed the community nurse to intervene on only two occasions when he might have become out of control. In recent sessions he has not mentioned attendance at the centre, as it has become part of his routine. Supportive psychotherapy has effected a change in his social environment. The last time he did mention the centre, it was to tell the therapist that he had supplied the centre volunteers with a recipe for cheese and potato pie, taken from his cooking class. Nine months of centre attendance had given

Erik the confidence to enrol in an evening class. The recipe had been used in the absence of the regular cook. 'I'm part of the team', he said. He was successfully relating to a new peer group, one which matched his level of ability.

☐ **Erik's care review**

It is important to recognise that failure in therapy is sometimes due to the therapist's neglect of the family's or other carers' needs. For carers to be successfully incorporated into supportive psychotherapy it requires that they be properly informed and counselled. They need to be instructed as to what to do and how to do it (Bloch 1981).

However, any meeting with a clients' carers or parents is likely to deprive the client of the therapeutically valid security of having found someone who will side with him against powerful and conflict provoking environmental figures. Not meeting with carers enables the therapist to form his or her own conclusion about the interrelatedness between them and the client (Fromm-Reichmann 1970). Explaining the question of distance as a therapeutic necessity arose when the psychotherapist was invited to Erik's care review by his key-worker. It was explained that, in order for Erik to feel safe in his sessions, it was important that the psychotherapist was not perceived as part of the organisation, and did not meet the other people who would be attending the review, including his parents. It was for this reason that the psychotherapist never visited Botley House or King's Hill Centre when it was known that Erik would be there. Erik talks freely about significant others in sessions as he perceives that the therapist is distant and separate from these people.

There remained the need, however to keep carers informed, and the care review provided a good opportunity to provide Erik himself with an ordered, concise account of his progress, on the occasion, coincidentally, of the first anniversary of the start of treatment. Erik had cancelled the session the week prior to his review, saying he wanted a break, so the psychotherapist did not have the opportunity to discuss any contribution the therapist might make to his review with Erik. The matter was raised with the therapist's supervisor. The issue to be resolved was how to provide the desired information on progress in therapy to Erik and his carers without breaking confidentiality, and without having Erik's explicit permission to divulge anything at all. The solution which was identified was to write to Erik. As he does not read this meant that the written communication needed to be via his key-worker.

The facilitative effect of written summaries as an ancillary technique in group therapy has been described as being most valuable if they are honest and straightforward about the process of therapy (Yalom 1985). The summaries are based on the assumption that the client is a full collaborator in the therapeutic process and that psychotherapy is strengthened, not weakened, by demystification. It is also a contact between sessions. For reasons which were not clear at the time, Erik had broken off from therapy. He resumed after two weeks and the summary would revive the sessions and provide continuity. Finally, it was hoped that the summary would enable Erik to review significant events and convert them into constructive learning experiences. On the day of his review an envelope was handed to his key-worker with advice on the contents. Erik had approved this course of action. The psychotherapist had taken the step of visiting him for the first time at King's Hill Centre to discuss the letter with him, as he was not attending sessions. There were three letters in all, an explanatory letter for the key-worker and other people attending the care review, and two sealed envelopes for Erik containing the therapist's view of the relationship in one and the therapist's view of his progress in therapy in the other. He had the power to withhold this information from others and was advised to speak to the therapist about the contents of the second letter before discussing it with others. This arrangement, it was felt, met the needs of all involved and preserved confidentiality.

☐ The effectiveness of psychotherapy

How effective has supportive psychotherapy been? When the psychotherapist asked Erik how the care review had gone he said 'They told me I was much better'. The therapist knew this to mean that a significant reduction in symptoms had occurred, which could be evidenced by the lessening of incidents, and that this could be validated from incident reports compared with the period before the last care review and before therapy. Changes in the outside context which also contributed to the improvement were group art therapy and the support of the community nurse. Feedback is an important part of supportive psychotherapy and feedback which is constant in sessions ensures that Erik is aware that he is capable of sustaining, over a long period of time, a demanding relationship, albeit a peculiar one. At the outset of therapy, broken relationships were the cause of the symptoms. His management of this relationship has led him to numerous rewarding relationships outside, including those at the King's Hill Centre, and has increased his self-esteem. Further, it has maximised his social functioning to the extent that it was possible to finish therapy with no detriment to his new routines. Support has been effectively transferred to the centre and the dangers of dependency obviated.

☐ Group therapy – A further step toward social relationships

The important matter of terminating therapy would be decided between the client and therapist, with the latter taking the discussion to the supervisor, as were the other major interventions in treatments, such as activation of the referral to the centre and the written summary compiled for the occasion of the care review.

Periodic reviews with the supervisor are necessary during the course of treatment when such questions as the dangers of dependency, compliance with the therapist's recommendations and availability of the therapist between sessions can be addressed (Bloch 1981). In Erik's case it was felt by the therapist and supervisor that individual therapy could usefully be rounded off by group therapy (Foulkes & Anthony 1957), as he had stopped attending group art therapy. Low self-esteem, ineffective coping with stress, poor control over emotions and specific interpersonal conflicts, such as those between parents and child, are problems of Erik's that could be tackled effectively in a therapy group. His acceptance of and by the group at the centre seemed indicative of the kind of motivation he would need to join a therapy group. When the time came to make the suggestion, this motivation could be examined further, in the light of his reaction. However, it does seem to be a logical progression of treatment, the factor of belongingness enhancing and confirming the effects of the social group (Foulkes & Anthony 1957), his membership of which had been secured by the application of analytic supportive psychotherapy.

Erik has, through therapy, acquired a stronger idea that he is capable and that he can enjoy a greater measure of self-control, rather than be the victim of his environment. He has handed his carers a psychological handling procedure which will not, if sensitively used, cause him to feel damaged. Through his success experiences, his self-image can be one which now feels more suitable.

■ Conclusion

This case study illustrates that psychotherapy can be used effectively with clients who have a mild learning difficulty. It has many real outcomes in terms of improvement in the quality of life which the client now experiences. However, it can be seen that this approach to working with clients is expensive, as the client received psychotherapy on a one-to-one basis on at least 26 occasions. Given the outcomes of this intervention with the client and the initial presenting problems it could be argued that this was a cost-effective intervention. If the intervention had not occurred it is possible that Erik's behaviour would have deteriorated further, resulting in further damage to the self, staff and the environment. This may have led to an expensive out of county placement being considered for the client.

This approach could also be usefully utilised to work with clients experiencing other types of emotional problem, such as loneliness, or clients who have been abused either sexually or physically.

As this is a relatively new approach to working with this client group, much research work remains to be carried out in terms of its continued effectiveness when clients are no longer in receipt of psychotherapy, with further developments to consider its use with clients who have severe and profound learning difficulties.

■ References

Bloch, S. (1981). *An introduction to the psychotherapies.* Oxford University Press, Oxford.

Bloch, S. (1982). *What is psychotherapy?* Oxford University Press, Oxford.

Brandon, D. (1989). *Mutual Respect.* Good Impressions, London.

Cole, A. (1989). Groupwork with people who have mental handicaps. *Mental Handicap.* September.

Corney, M. (1986). A lost child lives on. *New Forum.* 21(6), 12–15.

Frank, J. (1974). *A comparative study of psychotherapy. Persuasion and healing.* Schocken Books, London.

Freud, S. (1934). *Psychopathology of everyday life.* Penguin, London.

Foulkes, S. & Anthony, E. (1957). *Group psychotherapy: The psycho-analytic approach.* Penguin, London.

Fromm-Reichmann, F. (1960). *Principles of intensive psychotherapy.* University of Chicago Press, Chicago.

Gardner, J. & O'Brien, J. (1990). *The principle of normalisation programme issues in developmental disabilities: A guide to effective habilitation and active treatment.* Paul H. Brooks, Baltimore.

Grunewald, K. (1983). *Emotional responses of mentally handicapped people. Report of the sixteenth spring conference on Mental Retardation.* University of Exeter, Exeter.

Holmes, J. & Lindley, R. (1989). *The value of psychotherapy.* Oxford University Press, Oxford.

Humphreys, M., Hill, L. & Valentine, S. (1990). A psychotherapy group for young adults with mental handicaps. Problems encountered. *Mental Handicap.* September.

McKenna, H. (1990). Treat with caution. *Nursing Times* 86(11).

Marler, R. and Carroll-Williams, B. (1989). Groupwork on life events and sexuality with adults living in a mental handicap hospital. *Mental Handicap.* September.

Observer (1988). *Observer* Magazine, 8 March.

Orgler, H. (1973). *Alfred Adler – The man and his work.* Sidgwick & Jackson, London.

Pedder, J. (1989). Courses in psychotherapy: Evolution and current trends. *British Journal of Psychotherapy.* 6(2).

Rowan, J. (1983). *The reality game – A guide to humanistic counselling and therapy.* Routledge and Kegan Paul, London.

Rutter, M. (1982). Psychological therapies in child psychiatry: issues and prospects. *Psychological Medicine.* 21, 723–40.

Rycroft, C. (1986). *A critical dictionary of psychoanalysis.* Penguin, London.

Salzberger-Wittenberg, I. (1970). *Psycho-analytic insight and relationships: A Kleinian approach*. Routledge and Kegan Paul, London.

Sinason, V. (1989). Psychoanalytical psychotherapy and its application. *Group for the Advancement of Psychodynamics and Psychotherapy in Social Work* 4(1).

Szivos, S. & Griffiths, E. (1989). Group processes involved in coming to terms with a mentally retarded identity. *Mental Retardation.* 28(6).

Yalom, I. (1985). *The theory and practice of group psychotherapy*. Basic Books, USA.

Chapter 8

A systematic approach to care

Tony Gilbert

■ Introduction

Different care planning systems structure different roles for those people
involved in using them, such as service users, support workers and
professionals. The functioning of any systematic approach to care is also
dependent upon the environment. Together, the structuring of roles and the
environment set constraints to the degree of meaningful participation which
a user will experience, the implication being that, in order to promote
meaningful user participation, changes need to occur elsewhere in the
welfare system, not just within care planning.

The discussion of care planning systems and user participation begins
with a consideration of O'Brien's (1986) service accomplishments and how
they might be used in the evaluation of a systematic approach. Different
types of care planning system and the roles they create for the service user
and service providers are considered. The issue of user participation and the
constraints placed upon this by professional power, whilst relating these to
the accomplishments, will be explored.

■ Using service accomplishments to analyse care systems

The framework of service accomplishment has been developed from the
theory of normalisation (see Chapter 1 for further discussion). It considers
five areas that are viewed as having an important influence upon the quality
of a person's life (Wilcox 1988). This framework also has an important
function in creating and maintaining the synergy of the care planning
system. This is especially so where a number of different professionals are
involved in order to cater for all the different viewpoints (each informed by

120

their own particular conceptual framework or model). To be coordinated there is a need for a common language. This is one of the functions of service accomplishments. Also, by focusing upon the system from the view of the individual user, this framework places the user at the centre of service development and evaluation.

The individual components of the framework are outlined below. However, before discussing these individual components it has to be pointed out that these accomplishments by themselves provide aims or overall objectives which a service must strive to achieve. Within this the accomplishments need to be broken down into meaningful objectives for the particular user. Therefore the service accomplishments should not be viewed as five individual statements to be achieved without reference to the other accomplishments. A process of negotiation must take place between the individual accomplishments as they each interact with the others. The aim is to achieve the maximum potential from that service for the individual user. Each accomplishment does not have a point rating or something similar to help the people making decisions. Rather, the principle of what the person would like to do with their life is of major importance. Where people have difficulty in expressing or communicating their wishes the idea of involving an independent advocate is introduced (see Chapter 4). However, this, like the idea of participation generally, is problematic, and tensions exist between this and the professionals who organise them, as discussed in Chapter 4.

The five service accomplishments have been developed by combining them with three dimensions relating to the life areas of residence, occupation and leisure to form a matrix. This framework, originally developed for the Welsh Office (Evans 1988), directs people to look at what are broadly considered to be the major areas of a person's life: where they live, what their occupation is and what they like to do with their spare time. The advantage of this is that it ensures that one particular life area does not dominate at the expense of the others. Therefore, within the systematic approach, the competing perspectives of the different people and professionals involved can be mediated through using such a framework which views the system from the perspective of the person using it. The service accomplishments are now considered.

☐ **Community presence**

This accomplishment recognises that people should experience everyday events by using the facilities available to them within the local community. This should happen at the same time as other people who live in that community are using these facilities. Segregated services or segregated events within local facilities are recognised as denying this experience.

□ **Choice and autonomy**

This accomplishment recognises that people have individual preferences within a whole range of life options. It is also important to the idea of individuality that people are not just the passive receivers of services. Therefore people should be involved as much as possible in all decisions regarding their life and should be supported in making choices between real options. This accomplishment also recognises the importance of individual autonomy to personal growth.

□ **Competence**

This accomplishment recognises the need for people to have the opportunities to develop the skills that enable them to learn and grow as individuals. It recognises the importance of being able to take part in meaningful activities, supported with assistance if necessary. See Chapter 6 for further information on leisure activities.

□ **Respect**

This accomplishment recognises the importance of being valued within one's network and to be viewed as a person with a positive status and a positive self-image. People should be encouraged to engage in high status activities and to present themselves in the most positive way. They should be encouraged to avoid presenting themselves in a way that leads to them being stigmatised.

□ **Community participation**

This accomplishment recognises the importance of people having experience of a range of different relationships (see Chapter 5 for further information). This form of relationship will vary depending upon whether it involves lovers, friends, family, neighbours or people in the wider community. People need to have the opportunity to meet others and to interact with them in a valued and meaningful way.

Systems themselves are not, by definition, perfect. Nor should any system be viewed as fixed, immovable or beyond modification. In this, care planning systems should be viewed as providing, by their very nature, constraints both on the ways people act and on the ways people think and feel. A system is likely to have both strengths and weaknesses. As weaknesses could be integral to the design of that system they could be very difficult to resolve.

Moreover, if the weaknesses of a particular care planning system are acting in a way that supports the roles of those that operate that system against those that use it, the motivation to make significant changes might not exist. Therefore in the process of evaluating a system it is important that the perception of its functioning is not constrained by the assumptions upon which that system is based in the first place. All systems are constructed, often by those that operate them, and as such can be modified, made obsolete or replaced by new systems.

■ Care planning systems

Two care planning systems that are presently in use or under discussion for use in services for people with learning difficulties are now discussed. The first system will be referred to as life planning (Chamberlain 1985). This will be taken to include a number of other care planning systems that show similar characteristics, such as individual programme planning (Jenkins *et al.* 1988) and individual plans (Welsh Office 1983). The second system is that of shared action planning (Brechin & Swain 1987). The focus for the discussion will be the aims of the respective systems, roles structured for the service user and provider within the system, the models of human behaviour which inform these systems and the links made between these systems and their environment within the wider systems of social care.

Life planning is a care planning system that provides a highly structured framework within which a process of identifying individual needs, prioritis-ing of needs, goal planning and objective setting, and monitoring and evaluation of actions takes place. The central focus of the system is the review meeting, which takes place at regular intervals of six to twelve months. The system creates two major roles. The first is that of the chairper-son of the review, who is charged with coordinating events that are under-taken before the review, such as booking a venue for the meeting and circulating a needs list to the key-worker, and with the chairing of the review meeting itself.

The second major role is that of key-worker, who is a person chosen for the role on the basis of his or her knowledge of the client and having regular contact with this individual. The role of the key-worker is that of gathering information for the needs list from a variety of people who know the client, identifying the major people concerned with the life of the individual and inviting them to the review. The key-worker also attends the review to support and put forward an unbiased view of the client's needs.

The other major contributors to the review meeting are the client themselves, a family member, friend or advocate, and the people who are responsible for the residential or day services used by the client. Other professionals are not required to attend the meeting unless they have a specific contribution to make. The system recognises that clients may need considerable support as they might find such a meeting daunting. Each stage of the system is supported by a series of documents which provide pointers, and which serve as a means of recording and monitoring progress upon the agreed actions. Where the failure to meet an agreed action or need is due to a deficit in the service this should be recorded and forwarded to the manager.

Life planning has been developed from a number of sources that have been influential in the care of people with a learning difficulty such as normalisation, individual programme planning, goal planning and systems theory (Chamberlain 1985). The aim of life planning is to look rigorously at the full range of a client's needs by adopting a viewpoint that looks outward from the individual themselves. Life planning is also informed by a principle that states that the identification and the meeting of individual needs is central to the quality of life of the person and of the quality of services they receive. A particular client therefore may receive a high standard of service but if this fails to meet individual needs then the service is not of a high quality. This is an important point and will be used again when discussing the idea of participation as a need, in the context of the quality of a particular system.

The life planning system draws heavily upon behavioural psychology and its development has been strongly associated with the profession of clinical psychology. This theory has been highly influential in the provision of a developmental model and the techniques to promote skills development, competency and behaviour modification for people with a learning difficulty. One of its major strengths has been in the breaking down of skills or behaviours into a series of clearly defined and observable stages. This has led to the availability of a range of assessment tools which can be used to enable the identification of needs. The life planning system, rather than advocating a particular tool, encourages the selection of tools and techniques appropriate to the particular client. These are often complementary to those used by other professionals, as it is probable that these too have been influenced by behaviour theory.

The strengths of the life planning approach lie with the clearly defined structure of the system and its coordination. This provides the system with the momentum it requires in order to move forward. The use of tools and techniques developed from behavioural psychology provides a range of tested instruments which provide the answers to questions such as what to assess, how to plan, and what to evaluate and monitor. Also, the identification of service deficits links the care system to wider systems of management and resource allocation that provide the system's environment. There are, however, a number of limitations and criticisms of this approach.

Firstly, the dominant influence of behavioural psychology has been criticised for the way it identifies needs, in that it tends to focus upon what professionals define as deficits in the person, either in terms of skill or behaviour, rather than issues such as human relationships. The consequence is that the client is compared with what is described as an image of able mindedness or of able bodiedness (Oliver 1990). This has the effect of locating the problem within the person themselves rather than in the person's social or cultural environment. This means that the emphasis will always be upon changing the individual person in order that he or she might meet deficits that are defined by others.

Also, as the same professionals are involved at all stages of the care system, there is a weakness that emerges from the way needs are identified and resolved. This arises from a tendency for professionals to define needs in terms relevant to their own background (Wilding 1982; Oliver 1990). The effect is that this limits the definition of needs to those that can be provided by that professional, and that the monitoring and evaluation are carried out in ways that fit the professional models or theories being used. The idea of quality in this system remains under the control of the professional concerned (Dowson 1990). It will therefore be the needs of professionals rather than the wants of the client that become central to the system.

The problem of the dominance of professional interests in the life planning system can also be seen in the roles built into the system itself. The review meeting, which is central to the process, is ordered and structured in terms defined by the professionals. It may be that there are only two or three professionals in attendance at the meetings, but the skills and knowledge essential to feeling at home in such a situation and of making one's point are more likely to be concentrated into the hands of these people (Humphries *et al.* 1985). The idea of supporting the clients does not ensure that the event takes place on their terms.

It has also been proposed that, should a client respond in a way that frustrates the meeting, then the client will be able to leave the meeting which will then carry on in the client's absence. The system appears not to be flexible enough to accept that the client may be recording an opinion that states that he or she does not wish the meeting to continue, or that they are in some way unhappy about the events that are taking place. This highlights the fact that within the life planning system the idea of participation has a low priority.

The final area of weakness concerns the identification of service deficits and the apparent resolution of this problem by referring it to the manager. This issue relates to the system and its environment. It has to be remembered that the care planning system operates within a wider system and structure of social care. The consequence of professionals referring deficits to other professionals or managers is twofold. Firstly, the deficit itself is defined in terms approved by the professionals and control of the knowledge of the deficit is retained within the professional/management structure. Secondly, the deficit remains individualised; that is it does not become politicised by being unified with other similar deficits experienced by other users. The effect is that these deficits fail to find a powerful unified voice within the plurality of interest groups that compete for resources in the political system of a modern society. This identifies how the dual role of welfare professionals as agents of both care and control (Walker 1988) becomes institutionalised through the systems they help to develop. This issue will be explored in the discussion of professional power.

☐ **Shared action planning**

The second care planning system to be discussed is shared action planning (Brechin & Swain 1987). This system, developed in the mid-1980s, is described as building upon the impetus created by systems such as individual programme planning, which are now argued as being inadequate. Brechin & Swain (1987) claim that the need for a new system to replace life planning results from the increased independence and the flexible living patterns that people are now experiencing in the community. This contrasts with the blanket provision of routine care, which is the focus of the earlier system. Shared action planning seeks to build upon the possibilities for self-determination and the new and changing range of relationships and experiences found in community living.

Shared action planning (SAP) retains some similarities with the previous system in that it has a clear structure and a set of forms designed to support and record decisions and agreements at each stage of the system. However, SAP involves a radical shift away from the professionally dominated system of life planning. Here the focus is upon the empowerment of the person with a learning difficulty, their parents, friends or advocates and the support workers, through a process of building and changing relationships. The central principle in this system is that it is not just the person with a learning difficulty that should change or modify their skills and behaviour. Rather, people should be involved in a reciprocal process of empathy, trust, respect, growth, development and change. The aim is to work together to find answers to the issues that concern the person in a way which both feels right and which works. This is achieved by building upon the skills, experience and knowledge the person already has rather than identifying his or her personal deficits. It is argued that this system frees people's thinking so that they discover new ways of approaching issues and new opportunities for growth.

It is within the structure of SAP that the radical differences from life planning become apparent. Rather than the system orientating around a meeting called and dominated by professionals, who prioritise needs and agree a plan to be implemented by themselves and others, here the central focus is upon the creation of a partnership between the individual with a learning difficulty, a support worker and possibly an advocate. These people then meet in a way and at a time and place with which they feel comfortable. Formal meetings can be arranged if these people feel it necessary. Also, the relationship with professionals is one where they are approached for help and advice rather than one where professionals control the system. Moreover, the influence of professionals is viewed as limited due to them not having developed a relationship with the person concerned.

Shared action planning begins with a focus upon developing an awareness in the support worker of the range and quality of conscious and unconscious aims they have in their lives. It is also seen as important that the support worker recognises the importance of pleasure in living and learning. Upon this awareness the system then seeks to develop the long-term aims and shorter-term goals that will give it direction. The focus for these aims and goals is wider than the previous system, which adopts an achievement orientated approach. Here a whole range of ideas about circumstances and opportunities, as well as skills, are included. The system also directs people's thoughts in the direction of the three life areas (residence, occupation and leisure) referred to under service accomplishments.

The process of assessment follows the generation of aims and goals rather than preceding it, as in other systems. The strength of this approach is that aims and goals are not limited by or restricted to the areas considered by assessment tools and the professionals that use them. Assessment is viewed as a two-way process of developing communication and understanding. Structured techniques have a place but are only a part of this process of discussion, negotiation, forming impressions and making judgements that takes place between the partners. This is followed by stages of schemes of action and action tactics which consider the development and implementation of plans.

Again the focus is upon partnership, with those people who interact with the person in his or her social environment being as capable of change as the person with a learning difficulty. Each stage of the system is supported by the development of a diary and specific forms which enable evaluation and monitoring. However, the evaluation of the system is made by the person with a learning difficulty and their advocate. Also, the records and diary are viewed as being owned by the partnership and confidential to it. Decisions over who will have access or who will be circulated with information are made by the partnership rather than professionals.

Shared action planning draws heavily upon a humanistic model of human behaviour as described by Rogers (1979). Rogers views life as a continuous process of physiological and psychological growth which he refers to as becoming a person (Rogers 1979). In this, the basis for achieving full potential is a process of knowing how you feel by overcoming repressed feelings that inhibit growth. It is important therefore for people to form relationships based upon an unconditional regard, that is warmth and respect for each other regardless of what the other person thinks or does. This ability to respond to situations in ways that represent how the person perceives them, rather than in accordance with a pre-set and often imposed set of rules, creates a sense of autonomy and freedom for the person. It is easy to see the influence of this form of thought in the idea of partnership contained in the SAP. However, SAP does not close the door to other perspectives and it recognises the contribution that can be made by behavioural approaches. It is therefore quite consistent with the overall aims of SAP to use a behaviouralist approach when seeking to reach a particular goal, as long as this is decided upon in the context of partnership.

The strength of SAP lies in its commitment to empowerment both of the individual and of the support workers and advocates involved with the person. All of these people can be viewed as lacking power and control in care systems such as life planning. In focusing upon empowerment for all those concerned in the partnership, SAP recognises an important consideration if true participation is to be promoted. This is that the support workers concerned need to experience genuine participation if they are to appreciate the importance it has for the individual (Hallet 1987).

Another important indication of the social distance involved in the relationship between individuals and the support worker is the use of the metaphor 'partner'. This implies an equal relationship based upon dignity and respect rather than control. On the other hand, the use of the terms client, professional, chairperson and key-worker, as in life planning, identify the basis of the relationship as being one that maintains professional distances between those involved, both staff–client and staff–staff. It has been argued that the metaphors used indicate other conceptions that each has of the other and as a consequence they determine the relationships between people (Sumarah 1989). However, people need to be aware that changing relationships and metaphors to those of a partnership does not remove the potential for a power imbalance between the individual and the support worker and advocate, due to the likelihood that the latter remain more skilled than the individual. There is always therefore potential for a power imbalance. In shared action planning this is likely to be more subtle than before.

The weakness of the shared action planning approach lies mainly in the relationship it has with the environment within which it would have to operate. In moving the planning of the care system away from professionals and the systems in which they themselves operate it breaks the control they exercise over the definition of both problems and solutions. The problem is now defined by the partnership. Professionals are approached to ascertain if they have anything to offer. This in itself has positive benefits for the individuals, as it moves the system towards genuine participation.

However, in reducing the vested interest of professionals it fails to address the problems this may present for people wishing to use the SAP approach. The changes in the relationship with the professionals are fundamental and they need to be encouraged and supported in the release of the control they presently hold. Unfortunately, SAP leaves the people who are the least powerful exposed, that is the individual and the support worker, without either warning or guidance over the reactions they may face. This naïvety is continued in the idea of details of the care plan being confidential to the partnership. This is a very positive suggestion, but it ignores the fact that many organisations are subject to both professional and political monitoring, and again SAP leaves those weakest in the power structure to defend its principles. The introduction of the idea of contracting under the National Health Service and Community Care Act (Department of Health 1990) further reinforces this problem for the statutory, private and voluntary care sectors.

Shared action planning fails to recognise the dual role of welfare as both care and control. The power relationships that have to be changed to achieve the new state of participation and empowerment are deeply institutionalised in the structure of the welfare system. Proposing SAP as a development of life planning implies that one can be substituted for the other. This is unlikely to be the case, as the environment in which it has to function is one which is growing increasingly incompatible with the principles promoted by SAP. The development of consumerist ideas in the provision of welfare is viewed as running contrary to the principles of empowerment and participation. This is due to each concept being developed within different ideological approaches, the former being a market-orientated approach, whilst the latter lies within a political approach. Recent research has identified the tensions between these two principles (Croft & Beresford 1990).

☐ Participation and professional power

The issue concerning the extent to which an individual service user is able to control the events that happen in his or her life is central to the issue of professional power. It is a debate that rests at the centre of relations between users and providers of welfare services in modern industrialised societies. It also needs to be recognised that these two issues are indivisibly linked, for any moves which seek to increase user participation will have the consequence of changing the relationship with the professionals involved. This can be seen in the discussion about the different care planning systems.

The question is, how do professionals work to improve user participation whilst they are conscious of their dominant role in the power relationship in which they are involved? To take a neutral stance is insufficient, as the theory of social role valorisation demands that positive moves are made to promote the image and competence of the individual (Wolfensberger & Thomas 1983). This theory also demands that service providers are conscious of the devaluing and disabling effects of their actions and practices. As some people with a learning difficulty are totally reliant upon welfare services, they often have the least resources, both financial and personal, upon which to draw should they wish to redress this balance themselves (Klein 1984). In fact, many of the people involved will be experiencing what has been described as having multiple minority statuses

(Oliver 1990). In this, it is recognised that a person may experience a number of different statuses, each of which is disabling or devalued, that together compound the lack of autonomy experienced by the person.

The dilemma presented above can begin to be resolved by returning to the discussion of service accomplishments, for here is the basis for providing synergy to the care planning system. These accomplishments can be viewed as a unifying framework which acts to focus and coordinate roles and practices. This is in order that the system has characteristics and is able to achieve things on behalf of the user that are above and beyond the sum of the individual parts. This kind of momentum needs to be created if the competing interests of professionals are going to be overcome. This is a necessary prerequisite to maximising the potential of the service to a particular individual.

The notion that service accomplishments can address the issues of participation and professional power requires explanation. It has been noted previously that there is a need to negotiate and strike a balance between the accomplishments, as they should not be viewed as exclusive categories. However, for the purpose of this discussion it will be viewed as being mainly the concern of three accomplishments, those being choice and autonomy, respect and competence. These contain important issues relating to the process of the individuals interacting with professionals, whilst the other two, community presence and community participation, are mainly concerned with outcomes.

Participation is considered as being important; as Richardson (1983, pp. 54–5) states:

> It is argued that where decisions are made by others on their behalf, whatever the good intentions, consumers can have no sense of personal involvement with them. Participation in discussions about their everyday lives is therefore fundamentally important to individuals' self-fulfilment as well as freedom.

Hence it can be clearly seen that affording individuals the respect that considers them competent to be involved in their lives is the way in which choice and autonomy are promoted. From this it can be argued that people have a need to achieve ownership over their lives through a sense of personal involvement, thus taking the issue of quality raised by life planning as being the ability of the system to meet the needs of individuals. This therefore requires that participation is paramount within meeting the service accomplishments.

The issue of participation is also discussed by Parry (1972, p. 26) who provides the following insight:

> Managing one's own affairs is in turn held to be part of what it is to be a human being and a humane society will be one which maximises the opportunity for participating in the decisions that affect one's lives.

The implication here is that non-participation brings with it a status that is less than human. This again highlights the importance of participation when one considers the tendencies within society to view devalued people, such as those with a learning difficulty, as having a status that is less than human.

Participation is, however, problematic. This is especially so where service users lack the skills, experience and opportunities to maximise their potential to exercise autonomy without support. Communication alone does not mean that the power relationship between users and providers has been altered. The potential for professionals to reinforce their power by using participation to further their own interests is one which all those involved in the care planning system have to be aware of. Calling upon the notions of the professional ethic in defence of not seeking to maximise participation or in defence of accusations of manipulation is likely to be met by scorn from groups which advocate with or on behalf of service users. As Klein (1989) points out, much of the documented failure of responsibility by professionals was as a result of either scandals or the action of researchers, rather than by professionals themselves.

In order to promote participation the issue of professional power has to be addressed. In order to do this its sources need to be recognised. The basis of professional power lies with the special relationship between the profession and the state. It becomes institutionalised within the hierarchy of practices that constitute the welfare services, which, as was noted earlier, has a dual role, that of care and control. The implication is that solutions to problems will be framed in ways that complement the existing policies rather than in ways that threaten or contradict them. 'As social problems become the concern of professionals, the professionals become involved in a problem solving domain where problems and their solutions are seen as technical rather than political' (Galper 1975, p. 92). This discussion may appear to be abstract and removed from care planning, but it is important to remember that most welfare professionals are either trained or employed directly or indirectly by the state. The process of individualising problems starts at the interface between the user and the direct care professionals, that is, within the care planning system. It is at this point that the process of viewing problems as technical begins.

If the argument is accepted that participation is to be one of the prime aims of the care planning system, then the question arises of how to to assess and evaluate the level of participation achieved. Richardson (1983, p. 72) indicates that this is problematic:

> The consequences of participation are highly unpredictable. One cannot presume results on the basis of either the intentions of the participants or the specific structures through which they are involved.

Richardson is indicating that neither the adoption of particular structures, such as care planning systems, nor the good intentions of those concerned, is enough to ensure that the maximum potential for participation is achieved. This difficulty in evaluating the results of participation is compounded by the fact that at the level of the individual it involves many subjective factors, such as trust and self-confidence.

A useful framework for analysing participation has been provided by Arnstein (1969), who refers to it as a ladder of citizen participation. In this she develops eight levels of power relations which are identified in three broad bands:

Citizen power	Citizen control
	Delegated power
	Partnership
Tokenism	Placation
	Consultation
	Informing
Non-participation	Therapy
	Manipulation

From this it can be identified that the relations based upon partnership, which shared action planning seeks to achieve, have the potential to offer a meaningful role for the service user. Those of life planning, however, appear to fall short of this, as there is not a central role and relationship created for the service user. Therefore the potential achieved can only be considered as tokenism.

Another means of increasing the meaningful involvement of service users in their lives has been self-advocacy or citizen advocacy (Carr 1987). Advocacy is concerned with user empowerment and both care planning systems discuss possible roles for advocates, but only where a particular service user has difficulties in expressing his or her needs. Moreover, the political significance of advocacy should not be under estimated. Crawley (1988) indicates that there has been a growth in self-advocacy groups (see Chapter 4); however, most of these groups have been concerned with practical or social issues. Oliver (1990) argues that this should not be viewed negatively, as many groups need to develop self-help strategies prior to dealing with political issues. These groups provide an environment where the confidence and self-esteem of users can grow, and from this situation be transferred to the care planning system. Where the individual requires a citizen advocate this advocate can be used to balance the power relationship by providing an independent voice that can express the user's interests. Again there is the possibility that the aspirations of users will find a voice outside of the control of professionals and managers. Also there is the potential that these advocates will join together with other service users to provide an articulate user voice, as described in Chapter 4.

The weakness is that the power and knowledge remain almost exclusively the property of professionals.

☐ **Care management**

With the advent of care management it is possible that the power and knowledge will become accessible to the clients. Following the National Health Service and Community Care Act (Department of Health 1990), the concept of care management is becoming a reality for service users. It is envisaged that care management will ensure that services are planned and resources allocated to meet specific needs of individual clients. This is an attempt to ensure that people receive the services they require. Conversely, this means that the current over-provision of services to some individuals will not continue. An example of over-provision is where someone resides in a hostel, when they may only need assistance with household management to enable them to reside independently.

The cessation of over-provision would free resources which could then be allocated to other service users. It is anticipated that social service departments will take the lead role in care management. Effective care management should include (Department of Health 1989):

Identification of people in need
Assessment of care needs
Planning and ensuring delivery of care
Monitoring the quality of care
Review of clients' needs

Thus the care manager will be responsible for designing packages of care and ensuring that the individual receives this. It is not the care managers' function to deliver the package of care themselves, but they are expected to identify potential providers who will be responsible for implementing the care. The client will then receive appropriate care, possibly from a variety of agencies. It is hoped that the care management approach will enable agencies to work collaboratively in a way which has not been achieved in the past (see Chapter 1).

It is the intention of the government to give clients a greater say in how they live their lives. This should go some way to addressing the issue of professional power. However, it is also the government's intention that resources should be targeted at those in most need, and it is stressed that provision will have to take account of what is available and affordable. This again puts the professionals in a position of power, as they control the limited resources. Consequently, the power base of the client has not changed.

The services the client receives will be based upon the assessment data. The problems associated with assessment include the issue that only the client's weaknesses and deficits may be identified; whereas shared action planning should prevent this from occurring, care managers are required to identify need and the client's preferences may become marginalised (Beardshaw & Towell 1990). Potentially, care management is a step forward in service delivery and in the provision of individual packages of care designed to meet the individual's needs. However, there are inherent dangers that this approach will remain in the hands of the professionals and the intention of providing clients with a voice will not be realised.

■ Conclusion

As was previously acknowledged in the discussion of shared action planning, the awareness of the possibilities for different lifestyles other than those decided upon by professionals is increasing, and care systems provide a particular focus for the promotion of meaningful user participation. At the present time professionals have the ability to instigate these changes. The challenge for them is whether they view their loyalty as being to the service user or the state. The consequence is that, as user demands grow (whether through self-advocacy or group advocacy), the failure of professionals to meet the need for meaningful participation will be highlighted and the result may be that users will reject the role of professionals completely.

■ References

Arnstein, S. (1969). A ladder of citizen participation. *Journal of American Institute of Planners.* **11**(2), 17–19.

Beardshaw, V. & Towell, D. (1990). *Assessment and case management. Implications for implementation of caring for people. Briefing paper 10.* King Edward's Fund for London.

Brechin, A. & Swain, J. (1987). *Changing relationships: Shared action planning with people with mental handicap.* Harper & Row, London.

Carr, S. (1987). *National Citizen Advocacy, resources and advisory centre.* National Citizen Advocacy, London.

Chamberlain, P. (1985). *STEP life planning manual.* British Association for Behavioural Psychotherapy, Rossendale.

Crawley, B. (1988). *The growing voice.* Values into Action, London.

Croft, S. & Beresford, P. (1990). *From paternalism to participation. Involving people in social services.* Open Services Project and Joseph Rowntree Foundation, York.

Department of Health (1989). *Caring for people. Community care in the next decade and beyond.* HMSO, London.

Department of Health (1990). *The National Health Service and Community Care Act 1990.* HMSO, London.

Dowson, S. (1990). *Who does what? The process of enabling people with learning difficulties to achieve what they need and want.* Values into Action, London.

Evans, G. (1988). *The standard matrix.* Welsh Office, Cardiff.

Galper, J. (1975). *The politics of the social services*. Prentice-Hall, London.

Hallet, C. (1987). *Critical issues in participation*. Association of Community Workers, Bristol.

Humphries, S., Lowes, K. & Blunden, R. (1985). *Planning for progress? A collaborative evaluation of the individual planning system in NIMROD*. Research report 18. Applied Research Unit, Cardiff.

Jenkins, J., Felce, D., Toogood, S., Mansell, J. & De Kock, U. (1988). *Individual programme planning*. BIMH, Kidderminster.

Klein, R. (1984). The politics of participation. In *Public participation in health* (eds R. Maxwell & N. Weaver). King Edward's Hospital Fund for London.

Klein, R. (1989). *The politics of the NHS*. Longman, London.

O'Brien, J. (1986). A guide to personal future planning. In *The activities catalogue: A community programming guide for youth and adults with a severe disability* (eds G. Thomas & B. Wilcox). Response Systems Association, Georgia.

Oliver, M. (1990). *The politics of disablement*. Macmillan, London.

Parry, G. (1972). *Participation in politics*. Manchester University Press, Manchester.

Richardson, A. (1983). *Participation*. Routledge & Kegan Paul, London.

Rogers, C. (1979). *On becoming a person*. Constable, London.

Sumarah, J. (1989). Metaphors as a means of understanding staff resident relationships. *Mental Retardation* 27(1), 19–23.

Walker, A. (1989). In *The state of the market: Politics and welfare in contemporary Britain* (ed. M. Loney). Sage, London.

Welsh Office (1983). All Wales strategy for people with mental handicaps. Welsh Office, Cardiff.

Wilcox, P. (1988). Life planning. In *Towards integration. Comprehensive services for people with mental handicaps* (ed. D. Sines). Harper & Row, London.

Wilding, J. (1982). Professional power and social welfare. Routledge & Kegan Paul, London.

Wolfensberger, W. & Thomas, S. (1983). *PASSING (Programme analysis of service systems implementation of normalisation goals)*. Canadian National Institute of Mental Retardation, Ontario.

Chapter 9

Therapy in relation to people with learning difficulties

Heather Yule, Frances Loydd and Caroline Carter

■ Introduction

Whilst the provision of care is changing from hospital-based care to community-based care, it should be remembered that the majority of people with learning difficulties live at home with their families (DHSS 1971). However, the state provision of care has meant that traditionally therapists have been employed to work predominately within the hospital or residential environment. Consequently, with the move towards community care there is a need for therapists to change their traditional working practices.

As people with severe and profound learning difficulties move into ordinary houses in ordinary streets (King's Fund 1980), they may require support from the multidisciplinary team in order for them to live as independently as possible (DHSS 1984). Many of these people also have additional special needs, such as physical handicaps or limited language and communication abilities, which require specific specialist intervention to ameliorate the potential adverse effects of these special needs. Thus therapists may find themselves increasingly working with people with severe and profound learning difficulties who have additional special needs (National Development Group 1977).

One of the new challenges faced by therapists is in relation to ensuring that they utilise integrated facilities to meet the client's needs whilst ensuring that the service principles of enhancing community presence and participation are achieved whilst increasing the client's competence (see Chapter 8).

People with learning difficulties may have special needs which require specialised therapeutic interventions which will be provided by a member of the multidisciplinary team. An overview of the role of the physiotherapist, occupational therapist and speech therapist who work with people who have varying degrees of learning difficulty will be provided. It will be seen that these professionals adopt roles which differ slightly from their colleagues working in more generalist services. Two case studies are provided to highlight how the therapists work together effectively as part of a multidisciplinary team. In addition to this, the case studies indicate how the therapists can utilise community facilities to promote client well-being.

■ Physiotherapy

Physiotherapists, whilst being employed by health authorities, actually work with clients in a variety of establishments, including special schools and local authority controlled day services as well as health care establishments. The physiotherapists accept referrals from clients, the consultant psychiatrist and other medical practitioners, from community nurses, community teams and managers of local authority day services.

Following referral, an initial assessment is conducted. From this a treatment plan may be recommended and discussed with the client and the key-workers and carers. Without the cooperation of these people there is little hope of a successful and speedy outcome to the identified problem. This cooperation is vital. It is these people who will work with the client to implement the treatment programme. There is little point in the physiotherapist carrying out some treatments on a daily basis. For treatment programmes to be successful they need to be implemented on a regular basis as specified in the treatment plan. Consequently it is essential that the physiotherapist spends time with the carers in order to teach them the skills required to implement the treatment plan.

Whatever the problems presented, it is the physiotherapist's function to maximise the client's physical potential within the potential of his or her learning difficulty. The majority of the clients can be classified as having severe learning difficulties with accompanying physical disabilities. These physical disabilities have always been the concern of the physiotherapist. The therapist who works with this client group will also have the opportunity to use his or her skills and knowledge in expanding the lives of those who do not present an obvious case of motor dysfunction. The diagnoses which the therapist may meet can fall into several categories, such as cerebral palsy and epilepsy. All the conditions which the therapist meets will involve varying degrees of functional disability which will inhibit the individuals from being able to be fully integrated into community life. Being accepted by society is difficult for everyone. Personal appearance is important to our society, and when people are forming impressions about an individual they consider such things as the clothing which the individual is wearing, the gestures used and the physical appearance. Therefore it is important that the individual with a physical disability can utilise a variety of strategies to minimise the effect of their disability and consequently be accepted by society.

Motor problems can quite markedly affect the progress of people who wish to develop a more independent lifestyle. These motor problems might be poor posture or inability to carry objects without dropping them. These simple skills are taken for granted by the majority of society, as these are the skills which are mastered at an early age as part of normal development. However, individuals with learning difficulties who have not progressed through the stages of normal development consequently have mobility and/or functional disabilities.

It is the role of the physiotherapist to try to fill in the gaps in a person's development in order that they can have the opportunity to participate more fully in work and leisure activities. Through the application of active and passive exercise regimes it is the physiotherapy service's objective to accomplish with the client physical integration; individuality; a positive image, role and status; capability and competence; and continuity, autonomy and protection of rights.

☐ Physical integration

Whenever possible the therapist works with the client in the most suitable venue, for example skills development activities geared towards athletic type events should be carried out at the local athletic ground. Other sessions require the smaller, quieter environment of the therapist's room or a person's home.

The therapist works with individuals, their carers and the general public to overcome the barriers of physical separation and segregation, such as prompting mobility whether it be indoors or outdoors, either independently or with some means of assistance. This is in keeping with the service accomplishment of community presence (see Chapter 8). The therapist is always striving to develop the client's confidence.

☐ Individuality

It is the client's right to have a physiotherapy programme developed which will meet their needs and so maximise their strengths, talents and personality. In order to accomplish the individual care plan, the physiotherapist should identify and communicate any shortfall in the service which may prevent the deliverance of the care plan.

It is important that any service received becomes an incorporated part of daily life and enhances the individuality of the client. This is in keeping with the service accomplishment of choice and autonomy (see Chapter 8).

☐ **Positive image, role and status**

The ability to communicate with the client is a vital role for the therapist. A therapy session may be one of the few moments in a client's day when they do not have to share time with anyone else. The therapist has the opportunity to interact closely with that person, talking, touching, moving them, and enabling them to explore movement and their environment. The physiotherapist must recognise that he or she is not treating a condition, such as cerebral palsy or hemiplegia, but a person who requires a multisensory approach to their care.

The physiotherapist, when considering the provision of mobility equipment, special footwear or appropriate clothing, must ensure that what is provided will enhance the self-image of the client and that a positive image of the individual is recognised by other people in the community. This is in keeping with the service accomplishment of respect (see Chapter 8).

☐ **Capabilities and competence**

The physiotherapist must discover the client's needs before therapy intervention can ever be effective. The assessment process is ongoing and can take a considerable time to complete. It is vital that therapists work closely with all levels of staff, parents or relatives in order to build up the picture of the client. The assessment will include reference to the client's physical abilities and also their functional abilities.

It requires considerable interpersonal skills and time to establish a relationship with clients who have severe learning difficulties. The establishment of this relationship is vitally important to the success of any treatment plan. The therapist has to be sensitive to the moods, gestures and methods of communication used by the client. The therapist is often confronted with many physical problems, and consequently priority goals must be set.

Goals should be jointly agreed with the client and with carers. These goals are broken down into small steps which the client can achieve. 'Practice makes perfect' is an important point to establish with people who are involved in 24-hour care. Nothing can be achieved by therapy programmes unless they are incorporated into the person's daily routine.

It is important to choose activities with the client which will be of benefit to the individual; for example, reducing spasticity in the upper limbs will facilitate the more normal function of the hands and arms, and therefore there should be a functional activity available for the client to participate in, such as combing their hair with a brush held as normally as possible, or holding a toothbrush to clean the teeth.

The physiotherapist has the skills to assist the client to experience more normal movements, executed with more control and coordination and more self-awareness and concentration. The practical application of learned skills is of great importance and every effort should be made to provide opportunities for practice. This is in keeping with the service accomplishments of competence, respect, and choice and autonomy.

☐ **Autonomy and protection of rights**

In therapy sessions the therapist should ensure that the client is involved in the decisions relating to their own life. In practical terms, the client may decide that either they do not want to engage in any activity at all or they show preference for one activity over another. These decisions must be respected by the physiotherapist, but that is not to say that persuasion is not used to gain some activity, as continuity in treatment is part of the way to gain results.

The physiotherapist should respect the client's right to refuse treatment, to protect his or her body and to take responsibility for his or her action, but with the consequences being communicated to all involved. This is in keeping with the service accomplishment of choice, autonomy and respect.

☐ **Social integration**

The physiotherapist can encourage the use of community facilities for physical activity and recreational use at the same time as the general public are using the facility. A positive relationship can be created with those individuals who are responsible for managing the local sports facilities, such as the sports centre, the ice-skating rink and horse riding establishments.

In working towards social integration, the physiotherapist also has a role in accompanying a client into town to look at the shops or to have a snack at a café, as is also the care staff's role. These outings assist in developing the client's trust and confidence in movement and mobility. By ensuring that treatment can occur within everyday activities, the physiotherapist is able to provide the stimulation and motivation required for an individual to gain new skills and further independence. This is in keeping with the service accomplishments of community presence and participation, competence, choice, autonomy and respect (see Chapter 8).

■ Occupational therapy

Occupational therapists assess and treat physical and psychiatric conditions as well as people with a learning difficulty. The therapist works with individuals in order to assist them to reach their optimum level of functioning and independence in all aspects of daily living and to maintain their quality of life.

The occupational therapist is trained to view the individual as a whole in relation to her or his environment. This is termed the holistic approach. Where there is a deficit of function, the occupational therapist aims to enable individuals to live to their optimum level in their environment. The deficit may be physical, psychological or developmental. Enabling people to maximise their potential may be achieved by the use of individual activity and teaching, group participation, provision of specific equipment and adaptation of the client's environment, as well as providing training and support to those involved in the day-to-day care of the individual.

☐ **Working with clients**

As with other professions, the occupational therapists assess clients to identify their specific needs. Following the assessment a treatment programme is established. This plan states the aims and objectives for the client. Time management is crucial to the activities of the therapist. One client may respond to treatment for six or seven minutes whilst another client would participate in treatment all day. The therapist may work with the client for varying lengths of time, according to need. On occasions, short-term intervention is required, whilst for other people the interventions will be ongoing. To achieve success in treatments the cooperation of other professionals, care staff and families is of supreme importance.

Occupational therapists become involved with clients to provide independence skills programmes, enabling clients to use their energies constructively and to develop their social skills.

Provision of special equipment in relation to promoting independence is also the remit of the therapist. This equipment might be special feeding equipment or special seating. Occupational therapists who are employed by the Department of Social Services are also involved in housing adaptations, such as provision of stair lifts (DHSS 1984). Developing the client's competence in all aspects of daily living is also a function of the occupational therapist. Whilst carrying out established treatment plans the therapist actively works to ensure that the service accomplishments are achieved (see Chapter 8), and that treatment occurs in environments which promote competence, community participation and presence.

☐ **Counselling**

In addition to promoting independence, the occupational therapist also provides a counselling service. Counselling is achieved by listening to clients without passing judgement on the information received, thus encouraging clients to accept their own feelings and views without causing stress in attaining standards set by others. This leads to an increase in personal strength and control, expanding the client's capacity to deal with other difficulties more effectively.

☐ **Holistic approach**

As therapists utilise the holistic approach, their role can be extremely diverse. Historically, the therapist was mainly considered as someone to keep people occupied during certain times of the day and never at weekends. This view has changed, and therapists need to be flexible and to work at times appropriate for the client and for the activity.

It is important to ensure that appropriate activities for each individual are chosen. Therefore it is important to know what you are trying to achieve. If the aim of treatment is to encourage an upright position and increase upper limb movement and tolerance, there would be little point in asking someone to complete a puzzle. This would lead to a hunched position, and it is not a large activity, so upper limb movement would be limited. Thought should be given to activities such as window-cleaning, which involves holding the cloth, the sponge, a sensation of water, carrying and bucket-filling. This would encourage large upper limb movements, and an upright posture. Other activities which would also achieve this aim also need to be considered, such as painting a wall, washing-up or putting items in a wall cupboard. It is essential to offer a range of activities to ensure that clients are given choice in the matter.

■ **Speech and language therapist**

The basic role of the speech and language therapist working with people with learning difficulties is the enhancement of communication. A mission statement of the speech and language therapy service could be to provide a comprehensive speech therapy service to meet the needs of all people with disorders of communication, and to develop, remediate and maximise their potential communication skills.

For clients with learning difficulties this involves not only maximising the communication skills of the person involved, but also looking at the client's communication environment and the communication skills of his or her carers. Hence much of the therapist's time is spent on staff training as well as working directly with individual clients.

☐ **Assessment**

The form the assessment takes depends on the nature of the request for therapy and the client's level of ability. It is important to adopt a holistic approach to each client; that is to consider the whole person and all the situations in which he or she has to function and not merely to look at articulation skills. Some clients are able to cope with formal assessments, such as norm referenced or developmental scales. These can provide a baseline with which to compare later test results, enabling the therapist to judge the efficacy of therapy. These assessments may look at verbal comprehension (the understanding of spoken language), expressive language skills, interactive social skills or pragmatic skills (the use of appropriate and relevant language).

For all clients, informal or observational assessment is essential. Ascertaining how a client functions in his or her own world often provides a more accurate picture of the client than merely stating his or her level of verbal comprehension. Information about the environment and how other people in it interact with the client can also be gathered, such as 'Are there people who want to interact with him/her?', 'Does the client ever have a reason to communicate with others?', or 'What type of response does the client receive if he or she tries to initiate communication?'.

Staff and or family questionnaires are useful to gain a picture of the attitudes and expectations of the people involved with the client. They also enable the therapist to compare people's perceptions of the client's performance in different situations and to see how similar they are to the therapist's own observations.

Liaison with other members of the multidisciplinary team is important at this stage. The occupational therapist may be addressing many of the client's communicative needs with a programme, and it is economical of everyone's time to consider how it could be extended rather than designing a new one. There may be a particular handling procedure for a client which needs to be taken into account when formulating a communication programme, or which needs to be amended to increase the client's opportunities to communicate. In both these situations the clinical psychologist and speech and language therapist would work together.

All the information gathered from various assessment procedures contributes towards developing a therapy programme. This could be client-orientated, carer-orientated or a combination of both.

A client-orientated programme will involve encouraging a client to take some degree of responsibility for improving his or her communication; for example, Makaton signs taught need to be used, and articulation skills need to be generalised. Specific individual or group teaching/therapy may be required, or the therapist may choose to develop the client's communication skills via natural teaching within the client's daily routine. Skills acquired in this manner are more likely to be retained and generalised. Which strategy is chosen will be based upon the client's wishes and needs. The therapist has a responsibility to ensure that all carers understand the programme.

A carer-orientated programme may involve staff training, effecting a change in the client's environment or providing information about how to help clients generalise or use their communication skills. The client's environment, such as the carers who deal with him or her and the situations to which he or she is exposed, may be discouraging communication, such as in a home where the client's every need is anticipated and met. Nearly all referrals to the therapist necessitate a combination of client- and carer-orientated approach.

When a programme has been implemented, a review date will be agreed by all the people concerned. Success achieved and difficulties encountered can be discussed and the next stage of intervention planned.

The therapist also teaches new staff about communication skills and the role of the speech and language therapist. Topics which may be addressed in communication skills training are: interacting with a client at a level appropriate to the client's comprehension abilities; the effect of the environment in increasing or decreasing a client's desire or need to communicate; how to maximise communication potential within the environment; listening skills; and awareness of both staff and client's use of verbal, non-verbal and pre-verbal communication. Specific training for key workers to meet the needs of clients in particular environments or with more specific needs is another area of training in which the therapist could usefully provide a service.

The therapist aims to maintain liaison between different establishments and staff groups, such as residential and day care facilities, to ensure that therapeutic approaches adopted are consistently applied and that skills learned are reinforced and generalised.

Two case studies are now presented to indicate how therapists can work together to ensure that the client's needs are met whilst causing minimal disruption to the normal day-to-day process of living.

□ **Michael**

Michael is a young man who has spent the majority of his 24 years in a large institution for people with learning difficulties. Recently he was transferred to a much smaller unit where he shares his home with a small group of people. He now has the opportunity to benefit from a much more individualised programme of care.

Michael has a right hemiplegia, but is able to walk around independently. He requires a great deal of assistance in performing all personal activities of daily living, such as dressing, washing and going to the toilet. Michael does not have any verbal communication skills, but can often indicate certain needs by taking the staff by the hand and escorting them towards his want.

After allowing a short period of time to allow Michael to settle into his new care environment, an initial care review was requested by the person in charge. This review requested assessments from the physiotherapist, occupational therapist and speech and language therapist.

Over the following six weeks, each therapist made their own assessment of Michael's capabilities in close cooperation with Michael and the key-worker.

The occupational therapist addressed the areas of daily living. These were broken down into two main areas:

1. Personal activities of daily living, such as bathing, dressing, combing hair, going to the toilet, eating a meal and so on.

2. Domestic skills, such as making beds, clearing the table.

The physiotherapist addressed needs in relation to gross motor functions, such as the quality of Michael's walking, his physical ability to use stairs, to rise up off the floor and to move himself in bed.

The speech and language therapist liaised closely with Michael, the key-workers and staff to incorporate a non-verbal communication system into Michael's daily activities. This included the need to ensure that staff spoke to Michael at an appropriate level, whilst ensuring that the language used remained age-appropriate.

At a second meeting, six weeks later, the therapists, key-worker and other relevant members of the multidisciplinary team met to propose a package of activities for Michael. This package of activities had been agreed with Michael and incorporated a range of activities which he enjoyed.

The assessment data indicated a need for an integrated multisensory approach which would incorporate working with touch, textures, vision and sound. Michael would also be given the opportunity to develop greater body awareness, greater general mobility, and consequently improved posture and self-image.

It was agreed with Michael that he should attend the local day centre on a daily basis. His day was designed to include both individual and group work. This work was to be carried out in environments which allowed him every opportunity to concentrate, without being distracted from the task in hand by loud noise, too much movement of other people, or interruptions into the activity area. Some of the work would be carried out in environments that ensured community presence.

His individual occupational therapy session lasted approximately one hour a day. During this time he was introduced to activities which promoted the multisensory approach.

Cooking sessions introduced Michael to different textures when mixing ingredients together, for example flour with margarine. He could smell the freshly baked cakes when they were removed from the oven. At every stage, Michael participated to his maximum potential.

Community presence was achieved as this activity occurred in the local adult education establishment.

Clay work also introduced further smells, texture, colour and taste to Michael. He was able to explore the concept of weight, size and shape through this medium. As with all activities, he was in the situation to expand his awareness of his own body movements, an important concept which must be conscientiously pursued in order to progress activity achievements.

Michael was required to dress appropriately for his sessions, such as wearing protective clothing. Physical and verbal prompting were required initially to remind him to put on and remove this clothing. Gradually this has reduced to verbal prompting only. This activity also ensured community presence as it occurred at the local adult pottery for beginners course.

Computer programs have proved invaluable in developing visual scanning and communication through the use of different types of switches. Michael used the large flat concept keyboard on which two pictures of regularly based items were placed, for example cup and plate. On touching one picture on the keyboard he was able to see it appear on the screen. This activity occurred in the day service establishment.

The speech and language therapist worked with Michael to teach him Makaton. Instruction was also given to all staff in the most appropriate Makaton signs Michael should be encouraged to use to indicate his basic needs. It was important at all times when interacting with Michael to maintain conversation at a very simple but age-appropriate level; short sentences were used with physical signing when necessary. Over the last year there has been a significant improvement in Michael's comprehension and ability to carry out tasks.

The physiotherapy session involved activities to improve his posture and prevent any restriction in his range of joint movements. Utilising such basic movements as rolling and crawling his awareness of his own body became more acute. Whilst rolling, his whole body is in contact with a firm surface, with his own body-weight pressing into the floor causing increased sensation and more involvement in this activity.

Some activities which commenced as passive exercises became very active ones for Michael. He was delighted to find that he could make his leg swing in a sideways direction when his leg was suspended slightly off the plinth and supported in canvas slings.

The suspension activity was accompanied by ensuring the swinging motions followed the rhythm of Michael's favourite pop record. His facial expression indicated that he knew he was experiencing something new which gave him a good and satisfying feeling. These activities occurred in the physiotherapy department, which is where the majority of people receive their physiotherapy.

Hydrotherapy sessions provided him with another sensory medium. Over the last six months his ability to maintain his balance in the water has improved. Initially he would not stand unsupported and found himself being easily displaced by the pressure of the water acting all around him. He is now confidently moving around the water and splashes with his legs. This activity occurred in the local swimming pool, thereby increasing community presence.

Other activities in which he participated are weekly horse riding, sailing and gardening. His key-worker also takes him to the local swimming pool and to the pub at weekends.

Therapy programmes are carried out by day centre staff when therapists are not involved. It must be recognised that therapists work in close liaison with all other staff involved in Michael's care. Regular staff meetings ensure that programmes are evaluated and indicate the progress being made as well as providing an opportunity to plan ahead. Michael has developed more social awareness, is less tentative in his movements, will actively join in all sorts of activities with obvious enjoyment and is initiating communication.

☐ **Margaret**

Margaret is in her sixties and has been in residential care from the age of 16. Two years ago Margaret was given the choice of moving into a group home which she accepted. She has severe osteoarthritis in her shoulders and hips, which is progressively deteriorating. Margaret has always been clumsy and has poor coordination skills. Her verbal communication is limited and she has difficulty making herself understood. Margaret also has a hearing problem.

The occupational therapist was asked to establish a plan of care for Margaret. After assessment and discussion with Margaret and the care staff a number of areas were considered to have priority. The first was to monitor her mobility carefully; as this was decreasing, the physiotherapist was to be consulted. Margaret agreed with this proposal. Consideration also had to be given to her accommodation. The stairs became a problem, especially as there was only one toilet which was situated upstairs. Programmes to enable Margaret to transfer into and out of the bath were developed. New daily routines were established to take into account Margaret's reduced walking ability, and consideration as to the use of a wheelchair was discussed fully with her.

The speech therapist assessed Margaret's level of understanding, and a communication programme was implemented which enabled staff to help Margaret express herself more fully and clearly. Secondly, it was important to ascertain what Margaret desired in order to enjoy her life. She wanted to enter into social groups, such as an elderly person's club, shopping outings and cooking cakes. Although Margaret has not learned basic living skills, such as washing-up, these diminish in priority given Margaret's age. Activities which increase quality of life by providing enjoyment become dominant.

The occupational therapist provides regular supervision to the staff and Margaret's care plan is regularly reviewed with her. A crisis occurred for Margaret when she had a fall and was admitted into hospital. She received physiotherapy and occupational therapy treatment sessions from the community team whilst she was in hospital. This included walking short distances, activities to improve balance and outings to introduce her back into her routine. Margaret's self-confidence improved and a trial of a one-week stay back in the home was tried. This was successful, and Margaret was discharged from hospital. Occupational therapy input continued, with emphasis being on house alterations to construct a downstairs toilet and shower. The planning of bungalow accommodation may be a future necessity.

■ Conclusion

From the case studies presented, it can be seen that the therapists can establish collaborative working practices. This ensures that the client's opportunities for choice are broadened whilst maintaining their dignity and respect. This is achieved by the provision of activities which will enhance the competence of the individual, whilst utilising as far as possible ordinary community facilities, thus ensuring that community presence is achieved. This also provides the opportunity for community participation. By adopting flexible approaches to meeting needs the therapists can enable those individuals with severe and profound learning difficulties to achieve their maximum potential.

■ References

Department of Health and Social Security (1971). *Better Services for the Mentally Handicapped*. HMSO, London.

Department of Health and Social Security (1984). *Helping mentally handicapped people with special problems*. HMSO, London.

King's Fund (1980). *An ordinary life*. King Edward's Fund for London.

National Development Group (1977). *Day services for mentally handicapped . adults*. HMSO, London.

Chapter 10

Medical needs in a service for people with learning difficulties

Rosemary Baker

■ Introduction

In common with the rest of the population, people with learning difficulties also have many medical needs. An overview of the medical needs of this client group will be provided. It is beyond the scope of this chapter to provide a comprehensive treatment resource, but an insight into the special medical needs of this client group will be provided.

■ Historical overview

Historically, the care of people with learning difficulties was in the last century provided in hospitals. This has continued for the first two-thirds of this century. In the 1970s there was a shift in emphasis from hospital care to community care (see Chapter 1). Medical care in these hospitals has traditionally been under the supervision of a medical superintendent, and this person has usually been a psychiatrist. Indeed, all the consultant medical care of people with learning difficulties when they reach adulthood has been provided by psychiatrists. General practitioners have provided a supporting role in these hospitals, but their input has varied across the country. More recently there has been involvement of neurologists, neurophysiologists and clinical geneticists, but they have provided advice rather than being responsible for clinical care.

Although the consultants responsible for people with learning difficulties in hospital care have been trained as psychiatrists, they have usually had an overall responsibility for the medical care of these people. Also, as part of their training they have usually gained an awareness of the common physical conditions to which the clients were prone and of the interrelationships of these conditions with their mental and emotional functioning.

In fact, historically the roles of a consultant in learning difficulties and a consultant psychiatrist specialising in learning difficulties have been combined in the consultant psychiatrist in learning difficulties. With the advent of community care, many general practitioners have found themselves at a disadvantage, for they have not previously had much involvement with this client group. This has now been realised and a useful document has recently been produced by the Royal College of General Practitioners. This highlights the need for a continuing role for specialised expertise in the medical needs of people with learning difficulties in medical education at both an undergraduate and postgraduate level, as well as in other professions and disciplines.

The terms 'mental handicap' and 'mental retardation' remain the definitive medical diagnostic categories according to the criteria laid down by the International Classification of Diseases and the American Psychiatric Association's DSM-III-R (Talbott *et al.* 1988). Many people working in this field feel that labels and diagnostic criteria are not helpful, and indeed it could be argued to be positively harmful in that they could be seen as devaluing. Unfortunately, for the rest of the population they are necessary to provide a recognised structure for diagnosis and consequent treatment. This is the basis of the practice of medicine and can be argued of many other disciplines and professional approaches to care.

Traditionally, because the physician superintendent was responsible for the overall running of the hospital they were also responsible for the provision of other varieties of specialist input, such as nursing, psychology, physiotherapy, occupational therapy and speech therapy. This is now no longer the case, but with their lengthy training and experience as well as their working knowledge of psychodynamics it is hoped that consultants can provide a useful and necessary input into the professional team who are providing the specialist support for this client group. This role consists of information gathering and providing support to other team members and carers. In addition to this they provide specialised input from their medical and psychiatric training.

As the role of the consultant working in this service has changed radically in the last five years, and will probably change further, the components of the medical needs will be discussed under two main headings: the consultant in mental handicap and the consultant psychiatrist in mental handicap.

■ The role of the consultant in mental handicap

It should be stated that no such person has ever existed, except in the minds of referring agencies. This has been historically part and parcel of the all-embracing role of the psychiatrist working in the field. It is useful nonetheless to look at what is included in this role, for there is a very real danger that as the psychiatrist increasingly specialises in the psychiatry of learning difficulties both the knowledge base and the functions of this role will be completely lost. The function may be available for a short time, but as the present incumbents of positions are not replaced or are replaced by a new breed of specialist these skills will be lost to future generations of people with a learning difficulty.

☐ **Knowledge base and diagnostic expertise**

The first major component in the role of consultant in mental handicap is an in-depth awareness and knowledge of the various concomitants of the various syndromes associated with learning difficulties and how these might affect the behaviour of the individual.

An example of this is the evidence of thyroid disorder in Down's syndrome (Murdoch *et al.* 1977). Individuals who have Down's syndrome are especially prone to develop hypothyroidism; possibly because of an autoimmune response. It is actually very difficult to distinguish from many features which are associated with Down's syndrome anyway, so it is all the more important that it should be recognised and treated adequately. A study of individuals with Down's syndrome in Bedfordshire indicated that 30 per cent had thyroid antibodies, 7 per cent had gross hypothyroidism and 9 per cent had borderline hypothyroidism. This study also indicated that the incidence increased with age (Lobo *et al.* 1980). There is also an increasing awareness of the association of Down's syndrome and Alzheimer's disease. While there is no specific treatment for Alzheimer's disease, it is important that it is distinguished from hypothyroidism, which (as stated previously) can be treated; but of course it has grave implications for those providing care for the affected individuals. There are also a variety of other physical problems associated with Down's syndrome which can lead to behavioural changes and problems in management. These include congenital heart disease, the development of cataracts, and a defective immune system, which in turn leads to an increased susceptibility to infection and a higher incidence than normal of leukaemia. Also, as people with Down's syndrome age there is an increased chance of them developing epilepsy. This latter may be associated with the later development of Alzheimer's disease.

Other physical problems associated with specific syndromes include the development of epilepsy in tuberous sclerosis and the development of diabetes mellitus in the Prader–Willi–Labhert syndrome (Russell 1985).

Medical staff and others need to have an awareness that many people with learning difficulties have an altered pain perception. This, combined with communication disorders (see Chapter 9), can make diagnosis of problems such as toothache, earache and appendicitis much more difficult than in a person without these disabilities (Reid 1983). There is also an increasing need for specific diagnosis and recognition of genetic syndromes to give advice to families. This of necessity involves special investigations and time spent in research, as well as time spent with families.

☐ **Liaison with other medical specialities**

This should not be confused with the term 'liaison psychiatry', which has a wider meaning than just facilitation of cross referrals, including as it does the understanding and treatment of the psychological causes and sequelae of physical illness. This is not to say that people with learning difficulties do not have these problems. Indeed, they do, but they have a far greater need for cooperation and facilitation with the general medical and dental services in order to have their ordinary medical needs as well as their special medical and dental needs met.

Often special arrangements have to be made, especially for those people with severe and profound learning disabilities, to enable appropriate investigations and examinations to be carried out. This can mean arranging special times, special staffing support, appropriate sedation or a combination of these (Reid 1983). The same applies on occasions for operations and other in-patient treatments. Dentistry and occasionally chiropody are included here, along with the complete range of medical specialities. It would be helpful at this point to examine some examples to illustrate these points.

☐ **Tracey**

Tracey is a 22-year-old lady with severe learning difficulties and epilepsy. She has resided in residential care for ten years. She can speak in sentences, but does not do so unless prompted. Her epilepsy had been controlled by using phenobarbitone and phenytoin medication. However, this was changed to sodium valproate and as she then did not have any seizures for three years the medication was discontinued. She has had no further seizures and no longer takes anti-epileptic medication.

Tracey attended the local authority day care service. However, her behaviour became unpredictable and there were several aggressive outbursts. This was followed by a period of vomiting. Tracey was observed closely for a period of time. She did not return to the day service and her behaviour remained disturbed, with periods of vomiting despite the anti-emetic prescribed by the general practitioner. Tracey continued to have bouts of vomiting. On one occasion this was so severe it resulted in admission to the general hospital, where treatment to prevent dehydration was commenced. At this time she was found to be anaemic and this was also treated. Some months after discharge Tracey again started to vomit. In view of this history the psychiatrist consulted with a colleague in the radiology department. It was possible to arrange for her to have a barium swallow and barium meal. She was given the first appointment of the day and was accompanied by people who she knew well. The procedure proceeded without any difficulty.

The results indicated that Tracey had an acute duodenal ulcer and hiatus hernia with distal oesophagitis. This was treated with medication.

Tracey recommenced attendance at the day service and her behaviour reverted to its normal pattern.

☐ **Ellen**

Ellen also suffers from severe learning difficulties and Down's syndrome. She lives at home. Her behaviour has always been challenging, but it was reported by her mother and day service staff that it had become more disturbed than usual. Initially this was attributed to the change in routine, but Ellen's behaviour did not revert to normal after the new routine had been established. It was observed that Ellen's face looked slightly swollen and that she was avoiding eating biscuits. She was taken to the accident and emergency department by her mother where she underwent a dental examination. The dental registrar had great difficulty carrying out this inspection. However, it was ascertained that Ellen had at least one broken tooth. She was admitted for a thorough dental examination under general anaesthesia. It was found that she had two broken teeth and other dental caries. Dental treatment was given during the examination. Ellen's behaviour, although difficult at times, is much more settled than it was prior to this treatment.

☐ **Epilepsy**

One of the most important areas to provide adequate and comprehensive medical care in a service for people with learning difficulties is the treatment of epilepsy. A third of all people with learning difficulties eventually develop epilepsy. This is not really surprising, as it has an obvious association with structural brain damage.

Problems can arise in the diagnosis of epilepsy. This can occur because of communication problems where the individual may not be able to describe the aura that can occur as a prodromal sign of an impending convulsion. Also, a person experiencing a complex partial seizure originating in the temporal lobe may not be able to describe the unpleasant or unusual subjective experiences that are taking place. Incidentally, the person with poor communication skills will also have difficulty describing any side-effects to medicines which they may be experiencing. Epileptic motor sequences may not be recognised; they may be mistaken for stereotypical movements or other behavioural disorders. The next area of difficulty is in the actual treatment of epilepsy. Many people with brain damage are more sensitive to the adverse effects of medication. For some individuals with limited cognitive skills it is of vital importance to preserve what ability they have. Discerning the optimum level of anti-epileptic medication to achieve this and at the same time achieving the best level of seizure control so as to provide the best quality of life for the individual concerned can be very time-consuming and labour-intensive. There is also the potential for the therapeutic blood levels of anti-epileptic medicines to be interfered with by any other medication that the individual may be receiving such as anti-psychotics and antidepressants. Both of these types of medicines have the effect of lowering the convulsive threshold. In addition to this, the contraceptive pill interferes with any drugs which are metabolised in the liver.

When treating a person with epilepsy, especially if they have an added learning difficulty, the utmost care possible should be taken to preserve cognitive ability so that the individuals can continue to acquire skills and can realise their maximum potential for development.

■ The role of the consultant psychiatrist in mental handicap

The role of the consultant psychiatrist in mental handicap will now be explored. This was traditionally part of a wider role, but is increasingly becoming the principal area for medical specialisation.

□ Diagnosis and treatment of psychiatric illness

This, one might say, is the *raison d'être* for this medical specialism. When the closure of the large hospitals for people with learning difficulties began, it was stated that there was no evidence that this group of people had a higher incidence of psychiatric disorder, that there was no difference in treating it when they did have it, and that they were entitled to receive the same, albeit limited, services that were available to the rest of the population. In short, there was absolutely no need for this sub-speciality of psychiatry.

Much progress has been made in this area. Some of it has been painful, but there is now a general acceptance that there is a role for consultants trained in this speciality. Despite the obvious diagnostic difficulties, research indicates that there is an increased incidence of psychiatric and emotional difficulties in people with learning difficulties. In addition to this, their treatment is often far more complex and involved than in a person without such problems. This treatment can rarely be provided by the general psychiatric services available to the rest of the population.

☐ Incidence and classification of psychiatric disorder in people with learning difficulties

The recognised methods of making a psychiatric diagnosis by taking a history from a presenting individual and doing a mental state examination are often not possible with this group of people. Even if they are capable of understanding the concepts concerned, they may have problems communicating what they are experiencing for a variety of reasons.

People with mild learning difficulties can often give such information, and for them the same diagnostic criteria apply as for the rest of the population.

For those individuals who have more severe and profound learning difficulties it is, however, often possible to obtain a detailed history and descriptive observations form the carers of the person involved. In people who cannot communicate, the importance of this cannot be underestimated. Change of mood, change of behaviour and change of habit are all essential details in the diagnostic formulation of a person with learning difficulty (Reid 1983).

It is perhaps appropriate to use another illustration to show some of these points in more detail.

☐ John

John is a 20-year-old man who has severe learning difficulties. He is ambulant and has minimal self-help skills. He lived at home with his parents until the age of 17. He now resides in a small residential unit. John was referred to the consultant psychiatrist in mental handicap after an eight-week period of gradually eating less and less and having lost nearly one stone in weight. Physical illness had been excluded by the general practitioner. The symptoms which were noted by staff and elicited by the consultant by direct question were:

1. Sleep had been poor for about six weeks. John had been waking between three and four in the morning and wandering around the house.

2. John seemed less 'disturbed' in the evening and this was the best time to persuade him to eat.

3. 'Disturbed' behaviour. This consisted of being unable to settle. He had settled previously when he listened to music or did simple jigsaws, but this no longer happened. He was constantly wandering and was more preoccupied with his belongings, tending to constantly rearrange them.

It was established that John's father had been treated with antidepressants twelve years previously. However, he refused to discuss his symptoms and insisted he had been wrongly diagnosed. Other family members such as grandparents and aunts had also had a psychiatric history. This information was established when John's father had left the room.

Following the discussions with family and staff it was decided that John was suffering from endogenous depression, for which antidepressants were prescribed. Three weeks later John began to eat more and had regained half a stone in weight. He was also sleeping better.

■ Diagnostic procedures

There has been much recent work on diagnostic procedures in this group of people and on working out 'equivalents' to the recognised syndromes in the rest of the population (Collacott 1989; Reid 1989; Berney 1990; Fleisher 1990). This again highlights the necessity for continued work and research in this area. It is now widely accepted that there is an increased incidence of mental illness and emotional disorders in people with learning difficulties. The Royal College of Psychiatrists in a recent paper estimated that the incidence was as high as 50 per cent (Russell & Menolascino 1989). There are a number of reasons why this might be so.

(1) The first reason is the underlying structural brain abnormality or damage. Most people with severe and profound learning difficulties have major structural brain abnormality, and large numbers of mildly affected people also do so. Whatever the cause, it is well known that brain damage has an affect on behaviour, personality, language and intellectual function as well as on sensory and motor function, depending on the location of the damage, the developmental period at which the damage occurred and the nature of the damaging process. Brain damage also predisposes the individual to disturbances in levels of activity, irritability and to defective emotional and social control (Menolascino 1989).

(2) The second reason is that brain damage predisposes people to epilepsy, and there is now a wide body of research that indicates that the presence of epilepsy itself increases a person's vulnerability to psychiatric illness. A study conducted on the Isle of Wight indicated that of the total child population the overall prevalence rate of psychiatric morbidity was 6.6 per cent. Where children had an additional physical disorder which did not effect the brain the rate rose to 11.6 per cent, but where brain disorders were also present the rate actually rose to 34.3 per cent. A further study of two groups who both had brain lesions above the brain stem was carried out. One of these groups also had epilepsy, and the incidence of psychiatric disorder in this group was 58.3 per cent, whereas the incidence in the group who did not have epilepsy was 37.5 per cent.

(3) The third reason for increased vulnerability is the fact of the learning difficulty or disability itself. The learning difficulty is bound to have an effect on a person's lifestyle and ability to sustain interpersonal relationships (see Chapters 5 and 7). People with learning difficulties have to cope with the adverse consequences of being different and the social rejection this often leads to. They also have to cope with their perceived educational and performance failure. As children they will often find they are not able to play with or mix with their peers as equals. This is the beginning of lives denied status and satisfaction. As adults they will find it more difficult to gain employment and will find that leisure (see Chapter 6) and housing opportunities are often denied them. For various reasons, including financial disadvantages, they will not be accepted on equal terms by or with their contemporaries (see Chapter 6 on ideas to overcome this). Success in relationships is also often not achieved, owing to a combination of lack of appropriate skills and a lack of suitable opportunities.

(4) There is also a higher incidence of physical and sensory handicaps in people with learning difficulties and this can lead to various forms of sensory and learning deprivation which can also predispose to psychiatric pathology. By depriving people of opportunities the stigma associated with their difficulties is further increased.

Some conditions seem predisposed to problems. For instance, it seems to be commonly recognised that individuals whose brain damage was caused by the rubella virus *in utero*, which also often damages the sense organs, have a high incidence of a schizophrenia-like psychosis. This could be seen to parallel the paraphrenic illness which is often seen in the elderly with the onset of deafness and sometimes visual problems leading to a form of sensory isolation. Incidentally, it seems to respond to a similar approach to treatment.

(5) In some individuals these factors accumulate, and if on occasion there is a link with family stress and environmental limitations in providing care these can precipitate psychiatric or emotional difficulties. It is important also to bear in mind the consequences of treatment and the possibility of iatrogenic illness. One referral was in relation to an individual with obsessional drinking habits and face washing rituals. The cause of his problems turned out to be due to unbearable dryness of his mouth, which was caused by the massive amounts of drugs he was being prescribed and which he was unable to communicate to his carers.

Examples of the full spectrum of psychiatric illness can be found in people with learning difficulties, ranging from the psychoses and neuroses to personality disorders and adjustment reactions and other forms of behavioural disorder in response to stress.

Schizophrenia and 'schizophrenic equivalents' can be diagnosed. In people with mild learning difficulties hallucinations can be described. In people with more severe learning difficulties sometimes the positive symptoms are difficult to differentiate from any other type of acute behavioural disturbance, but the negative symptoms may be more easily recognised. Of course, apathy and social withdrawal can also be symptoms of depression, and physical illness may also need to be excluded before treatment can commence.

Affective disorders, ranging from depression to bipolar manic-depressive illness (including rapid cycling bipolar disorder) and anxiety can also occur. Many of the biological symptoms of depression can be observed by conscientious carers who notice changes in sleep pattern, appetite and general levels of activity. Also, subtle changes of mood can be noted, as for instance if an individual cries more or is withdrawn and not performing at their usual level. Similarly, levels of activity and obvious agitation can be observed in the manic or hypomanic person. Agitation can also occur in depression and needs to be differentiated from anxiety.

Anxiety can be very disabling, whatever a person's intellectual capabilities. Often the more able the person is the more anxious he or she becomes, particularly if pressures are constantly present to develop new skills and come up to the expectations of carers and professionals. Many quite able people with learning difficulties are referred for the management of anxiety which is preventing them from realising their potential.

As in all people presenting with psychiatric illness, a family history may give useful clues, as may the premorbid personality and any significant life events.

Personality disorders may occur in people with a learning difficulty, and like those of the rest of the population these are notoriously difficult to change. People with learning difficulties can also have psychopathic personalities. Even though they may be reasonably able intellectually this does not mean they are going to behave as they know they should. These people are capable of various criminal behaviours and are often quite aware of what they are doing and the consequences.

■ Treatment and management of psychiatric illness

Traditionally, all those who could not be treated in the community were admitted to the hospitals for people with learning difficulties. Often they were not discharged after treatment, although contrary to many people's assumptions, quite a lot were.

Now we do not have such facilities available everywhere. For the last five years people with mild and moderate learning difficulties with additional psychiatric illness who need more intensive treatment have been admitted to a general psychiatric admission ward. The criteria for admission have been that when well they were able to feed, clothe and wash themselves and were capable of going to the toilet unaided. Also it was understood that their place of residence before admission would be available for them to return to on discharge. These individuals have been supported on the wards by the community nurse, (learning difficulties) psychologist and other professionals. Occasionally it has been possible to admit people with more severe learning difficulties, but this has required supplementing the nursing staff both in numbers and in the relevant skills. It has been found that often the combination of a psychiatric illness with a learning difficulty produces symptoms and behaviour that are not seen in either of these conditions when occurring alone.

Those individuals with a more severe learning difficulty and additional psychiatric illness, together with some individuals in whom it is more chronic in its presentation, have to date been cared for in an eight-bedded unit. This unit was designed for people whom the services found difficult to manage in ordinary living situations.

■ Psychotropic medicines

The prescribing of psychotropic medication for individuals with learning difficulties generally follows the same principles as for the rest of the population, whilst remembering that individuals with brain damage are on the whole more susceptible to side-effects and there may be additional problems with compliance. Many individuals are extremely sensitive to any medication and may respond to minute doses, whilst others seem to be able to receive very large doses with little noticeable effect. As mentioned previously, psychotropic drugs lower the convulsive threshold and may interfere with the metabolism of anti-epileptic medication. This must be born in mind when prescribing treatment.

■ Challenging behaviour

Perhaps one of the most valuable contributions a psychiatrist can make today in trying to achieve quality of life and enable an individual with learning difficulties to maximise their full potential is in the area which is often referred to as 'challenging behaviour'. This term was first used in America by the Association for Persons with Severe Handicaps. It is important that the term is applied to the behaviour and not to the individual who from time to time may display this sort of behaviour. Challenging behaviour can include any of the following:

● Aggressive behaviour towards others such as biting, punching, kicking and scratching.

- Aggressive behaviour towards themselves (self-injury) such as head-banging, eye-poking and pica.

- Destructive behaviour, such as breaking windows and smashing furniture.

- Antisocial behaviour including smearing faeces, inappropriate sexual behaviours and screaming loudly.

There are many reasons why an individual behaves in these ways. It is in the analysis of this behaviour that there is an opportunity for all the previous subjects mentioned to be brought together, along with the more general psychiatric and psychotherapeutic skills acquired in higher psychiatric training, in a holistic approach to helping the individual concerned. This should be part of a multidisciplinary assessment of the individual's needs. This team should also develop and implement strategies for resolving the difficulties (Reid 1985).

■ Life events

Much work has been done in general psychiatry looking at the significance of life events in precipitating psychiatric disorder, and this work is also applicable to people with learning difficulties, who may have even more limited coping abilities. This also applies to the invariable transitions which they face in life as they grow up and includes the various developmental crises which we all face. These may be delayed and occur in a slightly older age group than that of the rest of the population. Stress has become very topical in the world of business executives and managers of industry, and is by no means exclusive to them. Stress is something that is also experienced by people with learning difficulties and particularly by their families and the people caring for them.

It is perhaps in this context of life events, transitions and stress that psychotherapeutic skills have much to offer (see Chapter 7). This approach is by no means exclusively a medical domain, but in the assessment and the ongoing support of staff engaged in this form of therapy a psychiatrist has a useful role to play.

■ Medical management of specific syndromes

Recent research has indicated that there is a specific role for the psychiatrist in dealing with self injurious behaviour and also in the medical management of some of the specific syndromes associated with learning difficulties

(Oliver 1989). Studies on individuals who have particular syndromes are now showing how biological processes may influence the development of personality, temperament and (consequently) behaviour. One of the best examples of this is the fragile-X syndrome but work has also been done on the Prader–Willi–Labhert syndrome, Lesch–Nyhan syndrome, Cornelia de Lange syndrome, tuberous sclerosis, Williams' syndrome and Down's syndrome (with its association with Alzheimer's disease, as mentioned previously), to name but a few.

In everyday practice psychiatrists work with colleagues from many other disciplines and backgrounds. To be clinically effective they must be able to collaborate with and complement the work of other professionals and be familiar with recent developments within the medical, biological and social sciences. They must also be aware of developments in a wide range of related areas, including education, rehabilitation, employment, medical ethics and social policy. Psychiatrists who work with people who have intellectual disabilities face particular difficulties, not only because they have so few colleagues in their speciality but also because there is such an enormous variety of needs in the people for whom they are providing a service.

■ Summary

The introduction of the impairment–disability–handicap model has done a great deal to clarify medical thinking about the ways in which disease processes have an impact on individual development. As more people with learning difficulties live an ordinary life in the community, so psychiatrists will need to assist general practitioners, other professionals, families and care staff to recognise emotional disturbance at an early stage and prevent the damaging consequences of an untreated psychiatric and/or emotional disorder.

Psychiatrists who have specialised in working with people with learning difficulties have much to contribute from their special expertise, but also have an important part to play in supporting other members of the professional team, families and other carers. They form an important reservoir of information, experience and expertise which needs to be effectively and efficiently utilised if these clients are to continue to take their rightful place in society.

■ References

Berney, T. (1990). Psychiatric aspects of well established syndromes. *Current Opinion in Psychiatry. Mental Retardation.* 3, 575–80.

Collacott, R. (1989). Rating scales used in the diagnosis and assessment of mental handicap. *Current Opinion in Psychiatry. Mental Retardation.* 2, 613–17.

Fleisher, M. (1990). Mental illness in the mentally retarded adult. *Current Opinion in Psychiatry. Mental Retardation.* 3, 603–35.

Lobo, E. de H., Khan, M. & Tew, J. (1980). Community study of hypothyroidism in Down's syndrome. *British Medical Journal.* 280, 1253.

Menolascino, F. (1989). Mental illness in the mentally retarded adult. *Current Opinion in Psychiatry. Mental Retardation.* 2, 594–602.

Murdoch, J. *et al.* (1977). Thyroid function in adults with Down's Syndrome. *Journal of Clinical Endocrinology and Metabolism.* 44, 453–8.

Murdoch, J. *et al.* (1977). Thyroid function in adults with Down's Syndrome. *Journal of Clinical Endocrinology and Metabolism.* No. 44, 453–58.

Oliver, C. (1989). Self-injurious behaviour: The lost cause in current approaches. In *Mental retardation* (eds V. Cowie & V. Harten-Ash). Duphar Medical, Romsey.

Reid, A. (1983). *Diagnostic problems in the mentally handicapped.* Medical Education International Ltd., London.

Reid, A. (1985). Psychiatry and mental handicap. In *Mental handicap: A multidisciplinary approach* (eds Craft *et al.*). Baillière Tindall, London.

Reid, A. (1989). Mental retardation. *Current Opinions in Psychiatry.* 2, 601–12.

Russell, O. (1985). *Current Review in Psychiatry – Mental Handicap.* Churchill Livingstone, London.

Russell, J. & Menolascino, F. (1989). Editorial overview. *Current Opinion in Psychiatry. Mental Handicap.* 2, 591–2.

Talbott, J. (ed.). (1988). *Textbook of Psychiatry.* American Psychiatric Press, New York.

Chapter 11

Education and training

Margaret Todd

■ Introduction

Much has been written in relation to education and training in terms of the underlying ideologies and methods which may be used to teach staff. This chapter does not have the scope to address all these issues and it is not the intention to reproduce this vast amount of information in a single chapter. The focus will be predominately on staff training as opposed to education, and some useful guidelines will be provided in relation to ensuring that required training is provided in the workplace.

As indicated elsewhere in this book, there exists a great need for a professional and skilled workforce to meet the needs of clients with learning difficulties. The need for staff development was particularly mentioned in Chapter 2 in relation to ensuring a high standard of service delivery and client care. Thus any service which is concerned with delivering quality care in a cost-effective way must incorporate staff development in its human resource strategy. Ensuring that staff development is given a high profile will also have the additional benefits of improving staff motivation and commitment, as staff will perceive that the employer is also interested in them as individuals. The issues surrounding education and training will be explored. In addition, the need to ensure that the staff receive the training required to enable them to perform the job which they have been employed to fulfil will also be addressed. This includes practical advice in relation to identifying training needs and assessing the individual's competence. The framework utilised links with the national vocational qualifications. The use of education as part of the process of implementing change is also discussed.

■ Education or training

Much debate exists as to whether any difference exists between the concepts of education and training. Education is taken as being a process of learning which is for the longer term (Curzon 1985). Education is concerned with the development of knowledge, values, interests, skills and critical ability, which will enable the individual to be more adaptable and flexible. As such, education does not have a fixed end-point but is a lifelong process of learning (Burnard & Chapman 1990). In contrast, training is seen as producing immediate results (Curzon 1985). Training is usually used when speaking of attaining predefined skills whereby all people undergoing training will end up with mostly the same abilities and skills (Burnard & Chapman 1990). Despite the very real differences which exist between the concepts of education and training the majority of people use the terms synonymously (Burnard & Chapman 1990), and thus they are used interchangeably in this chapter. However, the predominant focus is on training.

Regardless of whether the term education or training is used, the learning should be meaningful and useful. It has been stated that the ultimate aim of education and training is mastery (Curzon 1985). As the majority of staff employed to provide services to people with learning difficulties are currently unqualified, this chapter will focus on the national vocational qualifications, as this will provide the framework of training these staff in the future. Thus care will be delivered by either a professional or a skilled member of staff.

■ National vocational qualifications

The government established the National Council for Vocational Qualifications to improve vocational qualification by basing them on a national standard of competence which is required in the workplace. The council established a framework which is comprehensive and understandable. Its aim is to facilitate access to qualifications (National Health Service Training Authority 1991). National vocational qualifications are defined as a statement of competence clearly relevant to work and intended to facilitate entry into or progression in employment and further learning. National vocational qualifications (NVQs) will be available for all care staff regardless of whether they are employed by health, voluntary, private or social services. Currently two different types of NVQ are available to the care sector. These are health care support worker competences and residential domiciliary and day care competences. Both these competences are relevant to staff working with people with learning difficulties regardless of their employing agency. The level of competence currently available is at level two, but it is intended to develop this further to include level three and four competences. It is also the government's intention to mix both these competences in order to equip the staff with the skills they require. Currently, however, this exercise has been frozen due to the enormous changes which both the health and social services departments are implementing. However, a more cynical view could be taken about the cessation of this valuable work: that the professionals concerned may find that they could be replaced by a less expensive support worker, particularly as a level two competence for the residential domiciliary and day care service relates to assessing clients. Currently, only qualified practitioners are recognised as being able to assess clients. In addition to this the level three qualifications will indicate the ability to perform a wide range of activities including many difficult and non-routine activities which are appropriate to sustain regular outputs to the specified standard (National Council for Vocational Qualifications 1987). It can be seen that confusion over roles could arise (Pendleton 1991).

Competence statements contain specific standards in the ability to perform a range of activities which are work-related. They are written as outcome standards (see Chapter 2), and have assessment statements. The intention is that the training will make a measurable difference in terms of improvement to an individual's competence and that this competence can be tested against the national standards. The system takes into account on-the-job training that was previously unrecognised and is firmly based on job-related performance which is specified by the employer; that is, people will receive the training required to fulfil and meet the job requirements (National Health Service Training Authority 1991). Although people will be trained to ensure that they have the skills required to meet their current job requirement it will be possible for people to change their employer and have their competence recognised by their new employer. This is in contrast to the present situation. Currently, when staff change their employment they may not receive recognition for any on-the-job training they have previously undertaken. Many employers retrain new staff regardless of their skills, which may not be the most effective use of resources. With NVQs this will no longer occur, and consequently they will ensure that resources for staff development are used effectively.

To implement the national vocational qualification the procedure provided in Table 11.1 may be used.

Competence-based awards are structured in the following way (see Figure 11.1). Each contains a unit of competence which is broken down into elements of competence. The elements contain performance criteria and underpinning knowledge which the individual must have to achieve that unit of competence (National Health Service Training Authority 1990).

Table 11.1 Procedure to implement NVQs

Stage 1	Identify the skills required to meet job requirements.
Stage 2	Identify which units of competence meet these skills.
Stage 3	Assess the individual's competence.
Stage 4	Identify gaps in the individual's knowledge and competence.
Stage 5	Identify how these training needs can be met cost-effectively.
Stage 6	Estimate the cost of the training needed to meet the standards required.
Stage 7	Cost–benefit analysis, such as does the benefit of the individual acquiring the competence justify the cost.
Stage 8	Provide training.
Stage 9	Assess the individual's competence.
Stage 10	Accredit competence or go back to Stage 4 if competence not achieved.

■ Competence and national vocational qualifications

Competence has been defined as the ability to perform work activities to the standards required in employment (National Health Service Training Authority 1990).

Competence-based learning in the above framework is a move towards the student end of the learning continuum in as much as individuals work at their own pace and are assessed when they indicate that they are ready. The assessment occurs in the individuals' normal workplace. They are given credit for what they can do and get a statement of what thay can do even if this does not achieve the whole of the unit of competence. That is, they are awarded with those elements of the competence which they have mastered. It is up to individuals to provide evidence of their competence in order to be accredited with a unit of competence. In order for the system to work there need to be work-based assessors. With competence-based qualification people may not need any training if they can provide evidence that meets the performance criteria (National Health Service Training Authority 1990). That is, they will be given accreditation for previous experiential learning.

The assessor may not be able to directly observe everything, and there-

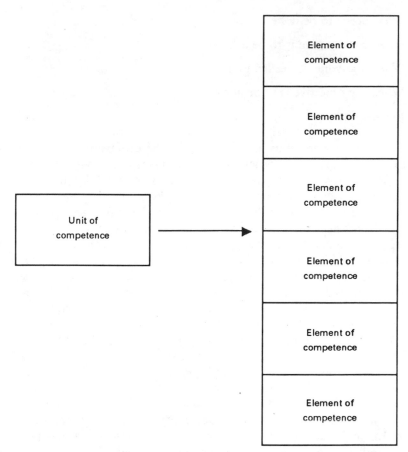

Figure 11.1 Structure of NVQs.

fore different evidence is needed, such as guided discussion with an individual, guided discussion with others, and review of existing records and documents which the individual being assessed has collected. Whichever method is used the evidence must be valid, that is it must be the right kind of evidence. It must be sufficient and relevant, that is appropriate to the performance. The assessor is expected to assist the individual with this development. The role again is towards the student-centred end of the continuum (National Health Service Training Authority 1990). Individuals should be involved in the assessment and encouraged to look at their strengths and weaknesses. This improves confidence and motivation. Targets and time-scales are reviewed and adjusted if they are not realistic. Training and assessment is discussed and planned. Assessors give feedback in a non-threatening way and a relationship built on trust and understanding is built up and maintained. The following areas are negotiated, agreed and recorded:

- What needs to be done.
- How the objective is to be achieved.
- Who, if anyone, is needed to help.
- When the objective is to be achieved.
- Review date.

Competence statements have been set by the professionals involved in the care sector consortium, such as social workers and nurses. The clients have not been involved in deciding what skills are required by the people in whose care they find themselves. Clients could be involved in the assessment of these carers, as they could be included in the discussion with other assessors' evidence, and this could be included in the quality statements of the organisation in their approach to total quality management. A statement of practice could be written to ensure that this occurs. This would go some way to redress the issues of professional power discussed in Chapter 8. Another issue which national vocational qualifications raise is that many clients receive care from unqualified staff, and when these situations occur the issue of who will perform the work-based assessment requires addressing. As mentioned earlier, it is the intention of the NCVQ that people will be assessed when they indicate that they wish to be assessed. It is unlikely that this will happen in practice. Employers will expect staff to achieve the number and level of competences required to fulfil the job requirements within a specified time. Thus if someone is employed in a post which requires level one competences it appears reasonable that employers will expect this individual to possess these competences within a pre-specified time period. The consequences of not gaining the required number and level of competences will become a management issue, and may result in the individual losing their current post.

■ Profiling

The decision about what competences are required is an important function of management. Managers must identify the skills required by post-holders in order for them to meet the job requirements. This can be accomplished in a variety of ways. Two methods are outlined below.

First, a manager can act as a facilitator to enable ward/house staff to identify the range of activities which they perform on a day-to-day basis. The skills required to perform these activities can then be identified by the group. These activities are then put on cards and given to each member of that team. They then write down the time taken to perform these tasks on a daily basis. These cards are completed in the workplace; that is each time a member performs a specific activity they write on the card. At the end of a pre-specified time period, such as one week, the cards are collected and analysed to ascertain which grades of staff are performing which activities (Wessex Regional Health Authority 1991). The analysis also enables staff to ascertain if highly skilled people are performing low-skilled tasks, such as the person in charge making beds. If there was a valid reason for the person in charge to perform this activity, such as teaching a client how to make a bed, then this would be identified and deemed to be an appropriate use of human resources.

This process identifies those tasks that do not need professional staff to perform them, such as routine ordering of supplies and stationery. This frees their time to spend with clients, which reverses the current situation whereby the professional staff spend less time with the client than unqualified staff do (Rosenhan 1973). Following identification of the activities performed by grades of staff and deciding which grade of staff should most usefully perform that activity to ensure the most effective use of human resources, job profiles or job descriptions are revised to reflect the change in content. The skills which are needed by each individual can then be matched to the available competences and appropriate training can be provided. As NVQs apply to all unqualified staff employed in the care sector, the staff groups should be multidisciplinary if other disciplines work within the house/ward.

Whilst this approach is useful in small organisations, it is probably too time-consuming in larger organisations, and it involves a high use of human resources. Therefore the second approach which could be used may be more appropriate.

The process utilised remains the same. However, each care environment is not fully involved. Instead, a sample of staff, which ensures representation from each grade and discipline, participates in the exercise. This approach is used across a care group or section of care groups. For instance, a group of staff from residential services would form one group, whilst another group might be formed from day services and a third group from ordinary houses. These groups could usefully contain staff from different agencies such as health, social services, voluntary sevices and the private sector. The major disadvantage of this approach is that it only provides a broad idea about the type of activity undertaken by each grade of staff and does not enable the differences in each care environment to be captured. The major advantage is that it is not as labour-intensive as the first approach and consequently may have a greater appeal to managers.

These suggested approaches ensure that the training required by staff is clearly identified. Where this cannot be provided in the workplace, such as when the underlying knowledge required about communications is to learn Makaton sign language, the manager can arrange for the appropriate training to be provided. This ensures that resources are used effectively, as staff will only receive training that meets their specified needs according to their job profile.

■ Assessment of competence

Assessment of competence is a key feature of the national vocational qualifications. Competence can be defined as possession of skills, attitudes and knowledge which enable the individual to perform fully in their role (Quinn 1988). The issue of who will assess in a workplace where the staff are wholly unqualified was raised earlier. There exists a danger that the most highly qualified staff will be spending their time teaching and assessing the unqualified staff. Whilst this should be carried out predominantly while participating in delivering hands-on care, such as by acting as a role model, there is a danger that this will not happen and that the qualified staff's contact with clients will be reduced.

Furthermore, where qualified staff do not possess the skills required to teach and assess in the care environment this will adversely affect the range of learning opportunities provided and consequently have a knock-on effect on the quality of care offered to clients (Kenworthy & Nicklin 1989).

Assessment in the care setting in both professional education and national vocational qualifications is criterion referenced. That is, a list of criteria for each competence is established and the individual is assessed against this. They either meet the criteria and are competent or they do not meet the criteria and are subsequently reassessed at a later date. Thus with criterion referencing the individual is not compared with anyone else (Quinn 1988). With criterion referenced assessment the question to be answered is 'Can this individual do a, b or c?' (Bligh 1981).

Unlike professional education, the individual undertaking national vocational qualification training does not have to meet the criteria within a predetermined time frame and can be assessed on as many occasions as necessary. They are accredited with those elements of the competence that they have achieved. Assessment is conducted on a continual basis; that is the criteria are assessed over a variety of occasions and situations and individuals are judged competent only when they can perform the skill in a range of appropriate situations. Continuous assessment ensures that a one-off performance on the day is not tested, as this performance may not give an accurate picture of an individual's performance over a period of time. A one-off assessment provides data that are possibly unrepresentative of the individual's behaviour and bears little relationship to their normal working practices (Quinn 1988). It is for this reason that continuous assessment is used, even though it is more time-consuming. Assessments can be used to monitor the individual's progress. This type of assessment is usually termed formative assessment (Bligh 1981). Formative feedback as to how well individuals are doing and what their strengths and weaknesses are is an essential part of the learning process. Thus assessment enables discussion to occur and is not something which is done to someone but becomes something which is done with someone (Harris & Bell 1986).

Unlike vocational training, professional education requires the student to acquire and demonstrate mastery of an increasingly complex and soph-

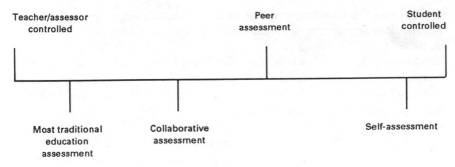

Figure 11.2 The assessment continuum.

isticated range of skills and knowledge as the course progresses (Kenworthy & Nicklin 1989). The interest of education is on the individual's continual development of skills and knowledge for long-term personal and job growth. As education is concerned with the future and the acquisition of skills for life, as opposed to meeting the immediate job role, norm referenced assessments are also used (Davies 1981). Where possible, the individual being assessed should participate in the process by the use of self-assessment, and this should form the basis for discussion on the final assessment.

Self-assessment is essential for students undergoing professional education. Self-criticism and self-assessments are fundamental to professional competence (Bligh 1975). People are usually concerned that students would overrate themselves. Whilst research indicates that students overrate their competence slightly, Bligh (1981) found a positive correlation between teachers' rating of students and students' self-ratings. If educationalists treat self-assessment seriously, then the students will also treat it seriously.

A problem with assessments is that all skills are deemed equally important when being assessed. This may not be the case. Few assessment schemes carry weighting for each element; however, this should not affect the quality of care. Clients could also usefully participate in the assessment of staff. Clients are the recipients of the care provided and consequently their views as to the competence of staff are a most relevant and important source of assessment data. Involving clients in this way would also assist in addressing the power relationship referred to in Chapter 8.

Just as teaching/learning can be placed on a continuum, so can assessment (see Figure 11.2). Collaborative assessment refers to discussion and negotiation by both the assessor and assessee about the assessment criteria and grading. This type of assessment cannot be used with vocational qualification training, as the criteria have been established nationally. Peer assessment either involves negotiation and discussion between the individual and a peer or assessment conducted by a peer. The use of peer assessment may overcome the problem mentioned earlier in relation to those situations where all the staff are unqualified. Self-assessment refers to individuals determining their own assessment criteria and judging their performance against them, or judging their performance against existing criteria (Harris & Bell 1986).

Mastery learning increases the likelihood that students will attain a satisfactory level of performance. People with low aptitude take longer to reach mastery of the skill. However, if they are given the time and feedback after assessment the individual will master the skill. Mastery learning is based on the idea that anyone can learn anything given the right circumstances (Davies 1981). In the practice setting, assessment is usually concerned with determining whether mastery has been gained. Feedback is essential as it helps the individual to identify how well they understand the subject and what errors they are making. This feedback must be corrective, deserved and respectful (Joyce & Weil 1986).

■ Education and change

Education has a vital role to play in the process of managing change (see Chapter 3 for change management strategies). One simple model of using education as part of the change process will be explored.

Pembury (1987) identifies five areas which need to be addressed when considering implementing change, regardless of how small that change may be. These are: creating the climate, planning, education, implementation and sustaining the change. This areas will now be considered in more detail.

□ Creating the climate

One person needs to be identified to act as a change agent. This person can be anyone, but it is preferable if it is someone who has the status to implement change, such as the person in charge. The change agent is responsible for communicating the ideas to others, gathering information, and eliciting the support of the staff concerned and other personnel who may be influential or affected by the proposed change. Thus, if it is the intention of the person in charge to introduce shared action planning it is important that this is communicated to all staff. In addition, other professionals will also need to be involved in the discussions, as power relationships will be changed as discussed in Chapter 8.

□ Planning

During this phase it is important to gain support and cooperation from all people involved. Identification of training needs is also important. Disseminating information and arranging a pilot scheme is also undertaken in this phase. Using shared action planning as an example to elaborate on this phase, it would be necessary to identify the level of staff's knowledge about shared action planning and the consequences of using this approach to care.

☐ Education

Having identified staff's training needs it is important to arrange for these needs to be met. It is essential that people have the necessary knowledge, skills and attitudes regarding the change. Communicating with and motivating others is also undertaken. Thus, if it is intended to implement shared action planning it is of vital importance that all staff receive the appropriate training.

☐ Implementation

It is important that everyone knows what they are doing, and therefore clear aims and guidelines should be provided. Thus the aim may be to ensure that all clients' needs are identified and met, utilising the shared action planning framework, by the first of the month.

☐ Sustaining the change

Even after the change has been accepted it is important to sustain it, as staff may try to sabotage it. Establishing supportive networks is one method of sustaining change. Thus establishing a weekly meeting to discuss the advantages and problems experienced using the shared action planning framework would sustain this change.

This simple model of using education to assist in the implementation of a change strategy should be useful to practitioners who wish to implement change in their area. The following is a practical example regarding how to use this strategy when implementing the setting of standards of care mentioned in Chapter 2, in the practice environment.

☐ Creating the climate

The person in charge wishes to set standards of care for practice. In order for this to succeed and be meaningful it is important that all staff concerned are committed to the idea. He or she discusses the idea at the team meeting to elicit support from the staff who will be affected and also discusses the idea with the immediate manager. The person in charge indicates the benefits of having written standards of practice against which performance can be monitored.

☐ **Planning**

The person in charge discusses the idea with all people who will be affected by the proposed change, including clients, their families and other professionals. During this phase he or she also ascertains the level of the staff's knowledge regarding writing and implementing standards. The cost of implementing this idea is also ascertained.

☐ **Education**

The identified training needs of the staff are met. This may involve the use of an external facilitator. The person in charge ensures that the proposed change remains high on the agenda and continues to communicate the benefits of the change to all concerned.

☐ **Implementation**

The person in charge draws up an action plan with time-scales for implementing the change. The people concerned know when they are to meet to set the standards, and they know the venue and duration of the meeting. The first meeting may be used as a brainstorming session to indicate those areas of practice for which staff would like standards. Subsequent meetings are used to write these standards.

☐ **Sustaining the change**

The person in charge ensures that the people concerned meet regularly to write the pre-specified number of standards. It is also important to ensure that staff receive positive feedback when the standards are monitored.

■ Adult learning

Research has indicated that where a human climate is created in the classroom, then more significant learning occurs (Rogers 1983). This probably holds true for the practice setting. Adult learning gives the ownership of the learning to the student. The teacher provides an environment which is conducive to learning. Thus in the practice setting the environment should be supportive of the learner. For adults to learn, the subject needs to be meaningful and useful. Adults learn more effectively if they are involved in the process (Brandes & Ginnis 1990). Adults need to know that the learning will be relevant before they undertake learning; that is, they need to know why they have to know it. Adults believe that they are responsible for their decisions and this needs to be reflected when they are in a learning climate. Adults are willing to learn what they need to know to function more effectively. Adults learn when the knowledge, skills, understanding, attitudes and values are placed in the context of practical application (Ogier 1989). Knowles *et al.* (1984) indicate that adults bring a wide range of experiences to their learning situation and consequently learn more effectively through problem-solving and experiential techniques. It is stated that adults are competence based learners in as much as they want to apply their skills and knowledge. Given this it would appear that vocational training will provide a successful training framework to meet staff's training needs, as it is concerned with skill acquisition. NVQs are based on behavioural objectives and as such are concerned with end products. Product is interpreted as measurable performance against the pre-specified behavioural competence (Pendleton 1991). It is acknowledged by the care sector consortium (Residential Domiciliary and Day Care Project 1989) that how people perform the skills is also important. The values people hold will affect how they carry out their role. Statements which incorporate values are classed as affective objectives and these are not included in the competence statements at present.

If the philosophy of normalisation is accepted (see Chapter 1) and care planning is based on service accomplishments (Chapter 8) and incorporates advocacy (Chapter 4) this would mean that employees require more than skills in order to deliver high quality care. Indeed, as the caring environment becomes more complex the acquisition of specific vocational skills may not be adequate to deliver the quality and type of care required and expected by society (Pendleton 1991).

■ References

Bligh, D. (1975). *What's the use of lectures?* Exeter University Press, Exeter.
Bligh, D. (1981). *Seven decisions when teaching students.* Exeter University Teaching Service, Exeter.
Brandes, D. & Ginnis, P. (1990). *A guide to student centred learning.* Basil Blackwell, Oxford.
Burnard, P. & Chapman, C. (1990). *Nurse education: The way forward.* Scutari Press, London.
Curzon, L. (1985). *Teaching in further education.* Holt, Reinhart & Winston, London.

Davies, I. (1981). Instructional techniques. McGraw-Hill, London.
Harris, D. & Bell, C. (1986). Evaluating and assessing for learning. Kogan Page, London.
Joyce, B. & Weil, M. (1986). Models of teaching. Prentice-Hall, London.
Kenworthy, N. & Nicklin, P. (1989). Teaching and assessing in nursing practice. An experiential approach. Scutari Press, London.
Knowles, M. (1980). The modern practice of adult education. From pedagogy to androgogy. Follett, Chicago.
Knowles, M. & Associates (1984) Androgogy in action. Applying modern principles of adult learning. Jossey Bass, California.
National Health Service Training Authority (1990). Work-based assessor resource pack. Health care support workers NVQ. NHSTA, Bristol.
National Health Service Training Authority (1991). Training performance measurement. A guide to some practical approaches. NHSTA, Bristol.
NCVQ (1987). The rational vocational qualification framework. NCVQ, London.
Ogier, M. (1989). Working and learning. Scutari Press, London.
Pembury, S. (1987). Achieving excellence through innovation. Nursing Standard Supplement. 2(10), 8–9.
Pendleton, S. (1991). Curriculum planning in nursing education: towards the year 2000. In Curriculum planning in nursing education. Practical applications (eds S. Pendleton & A. Myles). Edward Arnold, London.
Quinn, F. (1988). Principles and practice of nurse education. Croom Helm, London.
Residential Domiciliary and Day Care Project (1989). RDDC First draft standards. RDDC, London.
Rogers, C. (1983). Freedom to learn for the 80s Charles E. Mettill, London.
Rosenhan, D. (1973). On being sane in insane places. Science 179, 250–8.
Wessex Regional Health Authority (1991). A guide to reprofiling a workforce. Wessex RHA, Winchester.

Chapter 12
Summary

Margaret Todd

This book explores three major themes. The first is that of empowering individuals, various aspects of which have been discussed fully in Chapters 1, 4, 6 and 8. It can be seen that there have been many changes in relation to the delivery of services to people with a learning difficulty. Some of these changes have resulted from a change in social policy (see Chapter 1), and have become enshrined in legislation. Other changes have been influenced by events in Europe and America, such as the advocacy movement (see Chapter 4).

The issue of citizens' rights in the early days was predominantly focused upon minority disadvantaged groups. This has now become a key feature of government policy, and as part of this it has published a Citizens' Charter (1992). This charter will outline some of the rights of every citizen in the United Kingdom in relation to the quality of service the public can expect to receive. The influence this charter will have on people with a learning difficulty remains to be seen. As stated in Chapters 1, 4 and 8, whilst the power remains with professionals the effects may be limited.

However, the concept of service brokerage may overcome this. Service brokerage is a relatively new process in this country. It is a process by which clients can be empowered. This concept originated in Canada (Marlett 1989). Agencies employ brokers (care managers), who work with families to identify their needs and assist them in making appropriate choices as to how these needs will be met. The broker also identifies and negotiates individualised funding for people with disabilities (Brandon & Towe 1989). This is a key function of the broker's role and requires them to have good relationships with the client and family. With this funding the client purchases the services required. This system enables people with a learning difficulty to live autonomous lives in the community. The brokerage system also enables clients to act as their own care managers.

In the United Kingdom, service brokerage has focused upon reducing service duplication and achieving a set of goals agreed with the client (Glendinning 1986). The brokers have developed expertise in knowledge of the local services available for the client and regard themselves as the client's advocate (Pilling 1988). However, research has indicated that clients who received services from the projects which have used the UK version of service brokerage did not fare any better in terms of services received or the coordination of these services than the clients who received services from agencies who did not operate a service brokerage system (Glendinning 1986). This has been attributed to the lack of power the broker has on the service in terms of budget-holding (Challis & Davies 1986). This may be due to the fact that finances are tied up in providing traditional services. Consequently, funds cannot easily be released to be allocated to individual clients. If the Canadian system of brokerage was adopted the issue of advocacy and self-advocacy would become increasingly important.

People who are not able to speak for themselves would need advocates to ensure that they received the services required and to ensure that these services were of an acceptable quality. Chapter 4 deals with the issues of advocacy and self-advocacy in some detail. Chapter 8 addresses approaches to care delivery which may be used by brokers or care managers. The need to ensure that care delivery is in accordance with O'Brien's accomplishments is also discussed in the chapter.

It can be seen that services for people with learning difficulties continue to change, and the second theme of this book is that of enabling services to change. Chapter 3 focuses in detail on change management strategies. A framework for introducing and managing change is explored. This raises the issue of the importance of the need for a knowledgeable and skilled workforce. The focus of Chapter 11 is on education and training for staff. A useful framework for ensuring that staff have the necessary knowledge and skill is the staff development and performance review system. A variety of such systems exist. Regardless of which system is used the focus should be on the skills the individuals have as well as those areas that require improving (Torrington & Hall 1987). Historically, staff performance reviews have not been conducted as well as they should be, and this has led to staff perceiving the review as a potential disciplinary tool (Armstrong 1988). If managers focus on what people do well in addition to what they need to improve, staff may feel more satisfied with the process and may welcome this opportunity to improve their knowledge and skill (Torrington *et al.* 1989). However, this process places a responsibility on managers. If the manager has identified an area where the individual needs to improve, the manager then has an equal responsibility in enabling the individual to achieve this. There is little point in identifying weakness if opportunities for development are not given or are denied.

Change is perceived by many individuals as stressful, and ensuring that people have access to appropriate education and training is one way of lowering stress levels. There exist many other stress relieving strategies which are beyond the scope of this book, and consequently they will not be considered further. However, it is essential that attention is given to the stress which is caused by change when implementing a change strategy. To ignore this may lead to change not being fully successful or to the failure to implement the change.

The notion of quality is also incorporated in this theme. In order to implement the ideas outlined in Chapter 2, it may be necessary to develop a change strategy. In addition to this any change strategy developed will require monitoring throughout its implementation to ensure that the quality of the service is not adversely affected. The desired result of any change management should incorporate an increase in the quality of service provided.

The third theme of this book is that of working with clients in a variety of settings and, in some instances, in innovative ways. Chapter 9 explores how a variety of professionals can work together in a coordinated way to ensure that the client receives the required services. The importance of incorporating therapeutic activities into everyday experiences is highlighted and the focus is on enabling clients to participate in therapeutic activities which strive to adhere to the five accomplishments. This entails some blurring of traditional professional roles and a sharing of skills amongst the whole of the care team. The importance of working in partnership with client and carers is also considered.

This approach is further developed in Chapter 10 in relation to meeting the medical needs of clients. Some special medical needs are identified and the importance of carrying out a detailed medical assessment is discussed. The difficulties in carrying out such an assessment are also outlined and the importance of gathering information from the client and carers is identified. The medical approach advocated ensures that treatment will not diminish cognitive or physical functioning. This is an important consideration in terms of maintaining an acceptable quality of life. It is also important if the ideas outlined in Chapter 6 are pursued. This chapter provides a useful checklist to enable carers to assist clients to participate in a range of integrated leisure activities. Some of the activities identified are challenging, such as mountain climbing, and various research reports are cited. These outline the benefits of these activities to people with a learning difficulty, including those individuals with severe or profound learning difficulties. The findings reported are positive and will provide a challenge to carers if they decide to utilise these exciting activities to promote integrated leisure activities. A benefit of clients participating in integrated activities is that of developing relationships with other people. These relationships will be varying in nature and may range from acquaintances to strong friendship and possibly a relationship of a sexual nature. These issues are explored fully in Chapter 5.

Chapter 7 indicates the opportunities for staff to develop new knowledge and skills to work in a different way with clients. The use of psychotherapy for people with a learning difficulty may become an increasing necessity for the future to assist clients to cope with increasingly complex lifestyles. If clients require psychotherapy then they have a right to receive this from a trained psychotherapist. A great deal of psychological harm can occur if the client does not receive psychotherapy from a skilled and qualified psychotherapist. This is a challenging and relatively new way of working with clients in the future to enable them to lead satisfactory lifestyles.

This book is not a comprehensive text. It does not include all the relevant issues that require addressing when working with people with a learning difficulty.

Some major areas have been omitted, such as working with people with challenging behaviours, risk-taking, employment, and shared and joint training. Other areas have only been briefly addressed, such as care management, service brokerage, staff performance, and development review and assessment. The reader is encouraged to read further literature which deals specifically with the subject matter in greater detail (see Further Reading, p. 181).

It can be seen that the service provided for people with a learning difficulty is in a situation of constant change. Some of this change is generated by events external to service providers and some is a consequence of internal pressures. The professionals who currently provide the service will have a role to play in future service provision. However, this role may be somewhat different from their current role and individuals will be required to change to meet the demands of the service user and the community at large.

■ References

Armstrong, M. (1988). *A handbook of personnel management practice*. Kogan Page, London.

Brandon, D. & Towe, N. (1989). *Free to choose: An introduction to service brokerage*. Good Impressions Publishing, London.

Challis, D. & Davies, B. (1986). *Case management in community care: An evaluated experiment in the home care of the elderly*. PSSRU Gower, London.

Glendinning, C. (1986). *A single door: Social work with the families of disabled children*. Allen & Unwin, London.

HMSO (1992). *Citizen's Charter*. HMSO, London.

Marlett, N. (1989). *Independent service brokerage: Achieving consumer control through direct payment*. Walter Dinsdale Centre for the Empowerment of Canadians with Disabilities, Calgary.

Pilling, D. (1988). *The case management project: Report of the evaluation*. Rehabilitation Resources Centre, City University, London.

Torrington, D. & Hall, L. (1987). *Personnel management. A new approach*. Prentice-Hall, London.

Torrington, D., Weightman, J. & Johns, K. (1989). *Effective management. People and organisation.* Prentice-Hall, London.

■ Further Reading

Ashworth, P. (1986). *Care to communicate.* Royal College of Nursing, London.

Bachrach, L. (1990). Defining case management. *Hospital and Community Psychiatry.* 41(4), 454.

Beail, N. & Crook, S. (1987). Assessing knowledge. *Nursing Times.* 83(13), 50–1.

Billig, N. & Levinson, C. (1989). Social work students as case managers: A model of service delivery and training. *Hospital and Community Psychiatry.* 40(4), 411–13.

Bond, M. (1986). *Stress and self-awareness – A guide for nurses.* Heineman Nursing, London.

Bowman, G. Thompson, D. & Sutton, T. (1986). The influence of a positive environment on the attitudes of student nurses towards the nursing process. *Journal of Advanced Nursing.* 11(5), 26–8.

Brigden, P. & Todd, M. (1989). A way forward: Challenging behaviour in a day care setting. *The Professional Nurse.* 4(8), 377–80.

Brigden, P. & Todd, M. (1990). In search of the perfect assessment. *The Professional Nurse.* 5(4), 181–4.

Department of Health Study Team (1989). *Needs and responses: Services for adults with mental handicap who are mentally ill, who have behaviour problems or who offend.* Department of Health, London.

Goering, P., Wasylenki, D., Parkas, M., Lancee, W. & Ballantyne, R. (1988). What difference does care management make? *Hospital and Community Psychiatry.* 39(3), 272–6.

Hoefkens, A. & Allen, D. (1990). Evaluation of a special behaviour unit for people with mental handicaps and challenging behaviour. *Journal of Mental Deficiency Research.* 34(3), 213–28.

Hogg, J. & Raynes, N. (1987). *Assessment in mental handicap: a guide to assessment practices, tests and checklists.* Croom Helm, London.

Jones, R. & Baker, L. (1990). Differential reinforcement and challenging behaviour. A critical review of the DRI schedule. *Behavioural Psychotherapy.* 18(1), 35–47.

King's Fund (1987). *Project paper No. 74 Facing the challenge.* King Edward's Hospital Fund for London.

Krishnamurti, D. (1990). Evaluation of a special behaviour unit for people with mental handicaps and challenging behaviour. *Journal of Mental Deficiency Research.* 34(3), 229–31.

Open University Course Team (1985). *P555 Patterns for living.* Open University Press, Milton Keynes.

Open University Course Team (1990). *K668 Mental handicap: Changing perspectives.* Open University Press, Milton Keynes.

Wilson-Barnett, J. (1980). Prevention and alleviation of stress. *Nursing.* Feb., 432–6.

Index

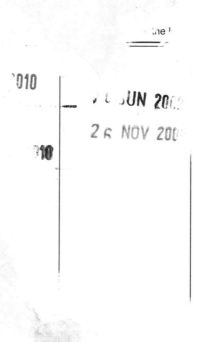

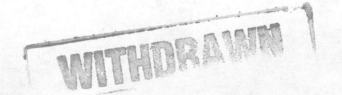